Also by Gail Sheehy

SEX AND THE
SEASONED
WOMAN

SEX AND THE SEASONED WOMAN

Pursuing the Passionate Life

Gail Sheehy

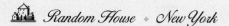 *Random House* ◆ *New York*

Published in the United States by Random House, an imprint of The Random House Publishing Group, a division of Random House, Inc., New York.

RANDOM HOUSE and colophon are registered trademarks of Random House, Inc.

ISBN 1-4000-6263-2

Printed in the United States of America on acid-free paper

www.atrandom.com

9 8 7 6 5 4 3 2 1

First Edition

Book design by Mercedes Everett

The photograph of Monika Bauerlein is by Robert Kelly. The photograph of Miranda McCloud is by Vic Losick. All other photographs are by Gail Sheehy. The illustrations are by Nigel Holmes.

To my sister Trish, a seasoned woman

Do I dare to eat a peach?

—T. S. Eliot,
"The Love Song of J. Alfred Prufrock"

Contents

Part III

Part IV

Part V

Part VI

Part I

And Now What?

*T*he idea for this book came to me in a dreamful state the morning my husband and I awoke on a mountaintop in Italy. It was a few days after I had put to bed a wrenching book about the families of 9/11, but already we were transported by the sensuous landscape of Italy's heartland, Umbria. Our window looked out on a mist-veiled gorge below the castle where a pope's daughter, Lucrezia Borgia, had been confined in the fifteenth century, six months pregnant, because of her promiscuity. Her lover later rode up the mountain and joined her there in time for the birth of their child. It was an arresting thought: a beautiful and sexual being who was a pope's daughter. Lucrezia was no longer young at the time of her imprisonment; and in fact, the pope soon after made her governor of one of the major territories of Italy, which she ruled ably from the castle fortress.

"I know what my next book has to be about," I murmured. "Sex and the seasoned woman."

"What's a seasoned woman?" my husband asked.

"You're lying next to one."

Like any *Aha!* moment, it seemed obvious once I began thinking about it. Before there was a worldwide hit TV series called *Sex and the City,* there was the mother of all female sex guides, called *Sex and the Single Girl.* A best seller in 1962, it remains a cult classic. The author, Helen Gurley Brown, was a trailblazer in the media by declaring that women are sexual creatures too, with both desires and career ambitions. She reinvented *Cosmopolitan,* which is still publishing sex advice forty years later. Helen, who employed me as a contributor to *Cosmo* in my early twenties, is still striking, still wearing her skirts three inches above her knees to parties she attends with her handsome husband.

Sex and the Single Girl helped spark the incendiary debate about women as sex objects versus women as people with equal rights and equal claim to their sexuality. Many baby-boomer women who fought those battles with themselves and others are now what I would call seasoned women, and they're still keen on sex. Significantly, 2004 marked the fiftieth anniversary of the publication of Alfred C. Kinsey's ground-shaking second book—*Sexual Behavior in the Human Female*—and it was that book, not his first volume on human male sexuality, that produced a vicious backlash that suppressed, even to this day, much of what he had tried to reveal.

"Sex" and "older women" used to be considered an oxymoron—rarely mentioned in the same breath. As late as 1996, the largest national sex survey since the Kinsey Report did not bother interviewing people over the age of 59. It was assumed that a woman's sexual pilot light was extinguished by menopause and she was content to slip into the desexualized role of on-call grandma and caretaker for whatever members of the family got old and sick first or whined the loudest. Even now, although there are glimmers of awareness in popular culture that suggest something a little more provocative might be going on, most women are still socialized not to expect much after 45 or 50—nothing much except dulling hair, corrugating skin, brittling bones, shriveling sex organs, and a social life centered around playing a little poker with the girls and maybe celebrating a birthday by tucking a dollar bill into the jockstrap of a male exotic dancer.

Do people really think we all trade the delights of touching and being touched for some hobby utilizing yarn?

Is there some inhibition ingrained in Americans that prevents us from imagining our parents—or, God forbid, our grandparents—between the sheets but not asleep? "What's amazing to me is not that older people fall in love and enjoy sex and feelings of attachment," says the anthropologist and author of *Why We Love,* Dr. Helen Fisher. "What's amazing to me is why Americans have never figured out that this is going on." Dr. Fisher, who has studied sex and love in more than fifty-eight cultures, sums up by saying that women today, having acquired economic power, have gained social and sexual power along with it.

"They're picking men from a wider range," she says "and they're doing it because *they can.*"

Before starting the research for this book, I, like many married women, had no concept of what the singles' scene was like these days for women in midlife and beyond. I got a hint one evening in New York. My husband was three thousand miles away, and I was hungry after seeing a play. At ten o'clock on a rocking Saturday night, the café across from the theater had no free tables. So I accepted a seat at the end of the bar, ordered supper, and pulled out my journal to make notes on the book just beginning to cook in my mind. I was deep in thought when the first young man's voice interrupted me.

"What are you writing, a book?"

"Maybe," I said. "I like to write."

"Okay, I won't bother you." But after a while, a second young man approached. "Why don't you write a book about me?"

I looked around the bar. It was chockablock with pretty young women with plunging necklines and Wonderbras to showcase their wares—young women apparently unattached. I asked the young men why they were wasting their time talking to me. They gave it some thought. I knew it wasn't my neckline—I was wearing a high-necked black T-shirt. It wasn't my shoes; they were sexy little backless numbers with a tiny heel (so I could actually walk in them), but they were hidden under my stool.

Finally the taller and handsomer of the two replied, "You look—interesting."

I continued chatting with the two young men, because, as I told them, I'd met my first husband in the White Horse Tavern.

"Your first?" they asked.

"I'm on my second."

They played along. "Then there's time for one or two more."

"Maybe, but it would be a close call. My current husband and I married after a whirlwind courtship of seventeen years."

They laughed. And then they told me all about themselves, which is what 25-year-old men always do. They tried to persuade me to write about them. "But you haven't told me anything interesting yet," I said. Then I listened, attentively, which is what 25-year-old women may forget to do. When I was ready to leave, they wrote their names and numbers in the back of my journal and asked me to call. Given the good fortune of a treasured marriage, I had no interest in following up. But I did walk thirty blocks in my backless shoes and never felt an ache in my arches.

I give you this anecdote not to brag (well, a little) but to point out one of the most welcome changes in American society. The ease with which these two younger men started up a conversation with me, and my own pleasure in engaging in repartee with them, began to open my eyes. The more I explored the concept of a seasoned woman, the more convinced I was that we are becoming freer of rigid age norms. At last, older women are shedding some of the stigma attached to age. And younger men, socialized in a postfeminist era, are more likely to appreciate a mature woman's independent spirit.

A great many women are finding "middlesex" more enjoyable than married life ever was in their thirties and forties, when juggling jobs, motherhood, and what's-for-dinner guilt made for mostly exhausted sex. Some remain married or have remarried, but, now freed from the long emergency of young motherhood, they are finding out how delightful it can be when it's about only you and him again.

In 2003, an English teacher from Berkeley published her boundary-busting account of sexcapades in late middle age. Jane Juska's *A Round-Heeled Woman* is her account of a year of hookups with dozens of different men who answered her personal ad in the highbrow journal *The New York Review of Books:* "Before I turn 67 next March, I would like to have a lot of sex with a man I like," it read. "If you want to talk first, Trollope works for me." She received a flurry of replies from interesting men and spent the next year having sexual adventures. After some thirty years as a celibate divorcée, she more than made up for lost time in her sixty-seventh year.

Unfortunately, too few women are enjoying their sex lives. In 1999, *The Journal of the American Medical Association* (*JAMA*) published a startling study finding that 43 percent of women aged 18 to 59 suffer from lack of sexual desire, pain during intercourse, difficulty in arousal, performance anxiety, or an inability to achieve orgasm. That's about 40 million women! (Thirty-one percent of men also admit to sexual dysfunction.) Perhaps most surprising, the problem isn't limited to any age group: Another study found that 36 percent of women with sexual dysfunction are younger than their forties; 32 percent are perimenopausal (in their forties and early fifties); and 31 percent are postmenopausal.

So aging alone cannot be blamed for cooling a woman's sexual fires. On the contrary, I will argue that it is the seasoned woman who knows best how to resonate with her sexuality. Today's women in their mid-forties, fifties, and sixties are at the peak of their lives. They consistently tell me—and other researchers—that they are happier and more productive than they have ever been before. Why? For one thing, women have a universal marker event to wake us up to the need to reexamine and revamp our lives: menopause. This natural milestone in the life cycle gives women a chance, even an excuse, to regather our forces and our energy, to seize the day, and to say, "This is the time to change."

On our day trips around Umbria to the lofty hill towns of Italy, my husband and I always found a terrace restaurant where we could sip a cool drink, hold hands, and lose ourselves in the magic of the moment. Inevitably, I noticed, there were other vacationing couples of middling age—husbands and wives, or lovers, who knows?—indulging in the same sweet pastime. I had a hunch that there was a lot more excitement and experimentation going on among women and men over 45 than our youth-obsessed society was aware of—or ready to admit. It was clearly time to extend my ongoing exploration of adult life stages.

Chapter 1

When Is It My Time?

*M*y first glimpse of what I came to recognize as a seasoned woman came in a chance encounter at an Oakland restaurant. A popular entertainer who was seated at the next table overheard me talking with my husband about my book. She leaned over to ask what it would be about. "It's about sex, love, and dating among women over fifty," I blurted out.

The entertainer's dinner companion rolled her eyes: "She's the poster girl for dating and sex after fifty!"

The entertainer, whom we'll call Bebe to protect her anonymity, was eager to elaborate. Bebe had been raised in the South with parents who were in love until the day they died. She had fully expected that she, like they, would marry for life. And happily, she had enjoyed an extended sexual honeymoon with the man she married in her twenties. It was in her forties that Bebe began to notice the cracks in their marriage. "But it's like you see a hairline crack in the wall in your California house and you say, 'Not to worry.' A couple of years later, you notice the crack is now a quarter inch wide—don't panic, it's a plaster thing. Then one big shake and the whole house tumbles down and you say, 'Wow, how did that happen?' "

In retrospect, she understands. Her frustration with her marriage was an echo of the complaint that fortyish husbands used before feminism went mainstream: "I've grown and, unfortunately, she hasn't." In Bebe's marriage, as in many more today, it was the husband who resisted taking risks to grow. It took her five years to get up the courage to ask for a divorce. She took that final step a few months before her fiftieth birthday.

"You must be crazy," she told herself. "You're going to spend the rest of your life home alone watching reruns of *The Brady Bunch.*" But it wasn't like that at all. Quite the opposite, she says; it's been the greatest adventure of her life.

The sociologist in me cast about for a context into which to fit this revelation. In fact, even while Bebe was settled into staid married life, a new public square of midlife singles was being flooded with divorced and never-married women and men. All the old rules were up for renegotiation. What was it like out there? I prodded.

In the first couple of years after her divorce, Bebe said, she had felt shell-shocked. "I went through a stage of mourning and learning to be alone. But people kept coming into my path. I met men at the airport, the grocery store, at church. Because once I started opening my eyes, there were really men everywhere. It wasn't like I was shopping, but they were flirting with me, talking to me, asking me out." Her therapist told her, "You have a neon sign on your forehead that blares: *Available.*"

"Pretty young women with firm bodies scared me as long as I saw myself as having to compete with them," she explained. "But what I found is I'm not in the same pool as they are. The older men who are looking for twenty- or thirty-something hard bodies are not the men who would look at me to begin with. These are two different universes."

Bebe's first dating experience turned the usual calculations on their head. He was a young man she met in church—and not just a little younger, *fifteen years younger* than she. "I was flabbergasted," said Bebe. "I was thinking, 'This gorgeous young man wants to go out with *me*?' " She bit the bullet and asked him, "Do you really know how old I am?" He said he didn't care. She told him anyway: fifty. He didn't seem fazed. He said she was smart and interesting and he just liked talking to her; he wanted to pursue it.

I asked Bebe if it was a revelation to her to have sex with somebody that young after living so many years with her husband. Her eyes danced and her voice jumped an octave.

"Oh, yeah! It was quite wonderful." Bebe quickly qualified her expectations. "I never looked at him as somebody I was going to spend the rest of my life with. I don't think he looked at me in that way, either. For six months we enjoyed each other's company and had a lot of fun. I believe people come into your life for a reason. He was the one who came into my life to say, 'It's gonna be okay, you can do this.' Getting over that hurdle was the big one."

Most of our grandmothers would find this a strange conversation. Half a century ago, there were certainly exceptional 50-year-old women who had lovers, and married people in their sixties and seventies who still enjoyed each other sexually. But it wasn't the norm. As the boundaries of our life span continue to expand in startling ways, the social definitions of age have shifted with the force of tectonic plates, altering just about everything.

Not all of us are as flashy as Bebe, nor do we all want to be, but I soon found that she is at the forefront of a trend. She is honest enough to admit that she misses some things about marriage. "When it was going well, we had great companionship." But like most women over 50 who can afford to walk away from a relationship if it has become a safe but hollow shell, Bebe savors her independence. She may have a neon sign on her forehead blinking *Available,* but it doesn't advertise *Looking for Husband.* She is looking for fun, companionship, maybe intimacy, but definitely satisfying sex.

❖   ❖   ❖

Sex and the Seasoned Woman is a book about a new universe of lusty, liberated women, some married and some not, who are unwilling to settle for the stereotypical roles of middle age. We are rediscovering who we are, or who we'd set out to be before we became wrapped up in the roles of our First Adulthood, when our primary focus was on nurturing children, husbands, or careers—or all three.

Millions of women today have struggled through all the predictable crises of their Tryout Twenties, Turbulent Thirties, and Forlorn Forties, and are bursting out into a whole new territory. Men, as they approach their fifties and sixties and start feeling the push to retire, often get a little shaky, wondering, Who will I be once stripped of the robes and powers of my position in the workplace? Women have changed robes so many times, they're ready to strip down and start fresh, feeling a boost of independence, exhilaration about what could lie ahead, and a surge of new powers.

What makes a seasoned woman?

Time.

A seasoned woman is spicy. She has been marinated in life experience. Like a complex wine, she can be alternately sweet, tart, sparkling, mellow. She is both maternal and playful. Assured, alluring, and resourceful. She is less likely to have an agenda than a young woman—no biological clock tick-tocking beside her lover's bed, no campaign to lead him to the altar, no rescue fantasies. The seasoned woman knows who she is. She could be any one of us, as long as she is committed to living fully and passionately in the second half of her life, despite failures and false starts.

Single boomer women like Bebe are not the only ones who are actively, even aggressively, seeking romance again, declaring their right to sexual satisfaction, and dreaming new dreams. Their boldness has caught on with "ladies" of earlier generations who were taught that their role was only to oblige their husbands and pick up after their children.

Margaret, an old friend and former radical who was still married to her only husband and living in rural New Hampshire, confided to me how shocked she was to hear stories from her contemporary female friends who are divorced or widowed in their sixties or seventies. "They're having romantic escapades with young guys, they talk about erotic discoveries, a couple of them have fallen in love again, but they want relationships beyond conventional marriage." Margaret still thought of herself as the free spirit who had walked the wild side in the 1960s. "I was the rebel, and they were the stick-in-the-muds. Now *I'm* the old married fuddy-duddy."

But you do not have to break up your marriage to change your life. Long-married women are also waking up to the possibilities of post-menopausal sensuality and proposing new contracts to shake the staleness out of their relationships and release their deferred creative energies. I met a California couple in which the husband had given up a stressful career as an attorney to help his wife pursue her dream: opening her own bookstore. Life partners who help each other feed and grow their passions can enjoy the magnified rewards of a marriage revitalized in middle life.

Counting Backward

Just how old is a seasoned woman? I define it very much the way Auntie Mame's friend Vera did when asked, "How old are you, anyway?"

"Somewhere between forty and death."

It's not over at 45 or 50, "it" being sex, intimacy, discovery of a new identity and a new passion in life. On the contrary, it begins all over again. Today, 50 is the start of a whole new cycle. You may have already lived an entire adulthood, but now you are at the beginning of another one—a portion of the life span that I identified in 1995 as our Second Adulthood.

Women's lives are long and have many seasons. As contemporary women, if we're healthy, we will likely be around longer than our mothers were. As I first reported in *New Passages,* epidemiologists say that a woman who reaches the age of 50 free of cancer and heart disease can expect to see her ninety-second birthday.

In our First Adulthood, we are consumed with just getting from A to B to C: pulling up roots from our parents, testing and proving ourselves as provisional adults, developing the capacity for intimacy, gaining the skills and credentials to support ourselves, and putting down our own roots. Given the prolonged American postadolescence—which for many middle-class women and men now stretches to the end of the Tryout Twenties—the First Adulthood today runs roughly from the age of 30 to 50. The years from 50 to 80 or 90 represent an even longer span. What to do with all the time left? People who try to hang on for dear life to what they had in their First Adulthood—the same dewy looks, the same high-energy job, the same steamy sex—may become their own worst enemies. A positive anticipation of our Second Adulthood allows for much less anxiety and greater flexibility.

A seasoned woman is not defined merely by her chronological age. Her inner image, including the ability to shed many of the roles that defined and confined her in earlier life, is equally important.

By the time you are 50, you have probably come to know yourself pretty well. You are better at separating possibilities from illusions. It's possible to learn to fly or start medical school or launch a cable TV show—we'll read about women who did—but illusory to assume that you can keep winning air shows or delivering babies or looking as foxy on TV as younger competitors. At some point you will probably want to change the emphasis of your work and take on the additional role of teacher, mentor, or guru.

Time is perceived differently after 50. People begin counting backward, thinking in terms of years left to live. But that may be forty years or more, and we can elect to make something magnificent of it. This is a huge cultural shift, making possible what I call the Pursuit of the Passionate Life.

When you stop to think about it, you probably know a seasoned woman who has embarked on a new life. Maybe it's an old college friend. Or perhaps it's your own mother and you're having a "Mom's run wild!" reverse-roles reaction. I've interviewed enough women whom I describe as WMDs—Women Married, Dammit!—to know that many wrestle with a rhetorical question almost as vexing as Hamlet's dilemma: *to leap or not to leap?* Is it nobler for a woman to stick with a stultifying marriage or better to step off into the unknown? Or perhaps you're widowed or divorced but not really "out there"—and wondering what it's like for women who do take the leap.

The Wild-Haired Years

The widow who first came to my mind was Peggy, a professor of political science at a prestigious college, whose story I told in *New Passages.* A flaming redhead with an infectious laugh, Peggy waged five years of a gallant battle with her husband, Chuck, against his prostate cancer. Once widowed, Peggy was forced to learn to be alone. Her first solo vacation she spent in the Canadian Gulf Islands, plunging into the chilly sea every morning at dawn and rising, refreshed and tingling with life, like Venus from the sea. "It made me feel like I could be a spicy woman again," she told me. "It's ironic. When nothing bigger can happen to you in a negative sense, you feel invulnerable. Since he's gone, I'm more *me* than I ever was. I dare more. My first question now is always 'Well, why not?' I call it my wild hair. When I don't have my wild hair, I'm sad. But when I have it, there's a certain elation."

After passing her sixty-fifth birthday, Peggy met an interesting man at a political rally. They saw each other a few times for dinner and conversation, though "having another romance was the furthest thing from my mind," she told me. "But one day the fun-loving Peggy in me picked up the phone on the spur of the moment and invited this man to go to Big Sur for a weekend. I thought, 'Well, why not?' "

When Jack pulled up at her house in his dashing black Lexus, Peggy was in jeans at her sink doing dishes. At the last moment, hearing her mother's censorious voice in her ears, she couldn't step over the line. She kept her hands plunged into hot soapy water and mumbled, "I can't do this, I'm sorry." Jack suggested that it would be just a relaxing getaway weekend. Peggy demurred: "I know, but we both know where this is going." Jack kept gently filibustering. She asked him to wait in the car.

"In a wild-haired moment, I grabbed the first thing I could find—a big black garbage bag—and stuffed some clothes inside before I could change my mind again." When Peggy emerged from her kitchen, Jack wondered, No suitcase? Had she chickened out after all? He just hadn't noticed what she was dragging behind her.

Jack laughed. He caught her spirit of spontaneity, and on their arrival at the exclusive waterfront inn, he handed the garbage bag to the doorman with a flourish. He watched with a sexy gleam in his eye as Peggy swept into the lobby with the light-footed grandeur of a duchess.

Less than a year later Peggy agreed to marry Jack, provided they both accepted an agreement: she would continue teaching, and each of them would keep their own home and sense of community. Peggy shifted her emphasis into creating reentry programs at local colleges for women who have been divorced, abandoned, or widowed and have to start over again, as she had. In their eight years together, she and her adoring new husband have traveled just about every continent and shared adventures. Most recently, they sailed the Croatian coast with Jack skippering and Peggy and her children as the crew.

The most indelible change has been in Peggy herself: she hasn't lost her wild hair again, not for a moment.

Chapter 2

The Journey Ahead

*W*hen I wrote *Passages* in the mid-1970s, I stopped parsing the stages of adult development at age 50. How quaint that now seems! I couldn't imagine then what kind of change and growth could take place beyond that sobering marker of middle age. And I certainly didn't envision love matches between Hollywood sex goddesses in their forties with much younger Adonises, as displayed by the trend-setting Madonna, who at 42 married a man ten years her junior, and by Demi Moore, who offered further evidence of this liberating new trend when she chose for her third husband the 27-year-old actor Ashton Kutcher.

Believe it or not, back in the 1970s "midlife" for women could begin in the mid-thirties. The years between 35 and 45 were the passage to middle age, when a woman had to pick up on any deferred dreams or settle for the bed she had made. Thirty years ago, I had only an inkling of the historic revolution about to shake up our social order: Americans were taking longer to grow up and much longer to die, shifting all of the stages of adulthood ahead by at least ten years. Now the mortality crisis that precipitates the midlife passage is usually delayed until somewhere between the mid-forties and mid-fifties.

The U.S. Census Bureau calls Americans "elderly" at 65. But in a major national poll of its boomer-aged members, the AARP asked a question that revealed the real mental image most boomers carry around in their heads:

"When will you be old?" Boomers said "79." They see themselves as in midlife until they reach the brink of their 80s.

In the year 2006, almost a million of the earliest boomer women will be ready to celebrate their sixtieth birthday. "Sixty is the new forty!" their friends will probably assure them. As boomers move into this new territory, they keep redefining it.

I remember TV diva Barbara Walters telling me after her daughter graduated from college, "Now I can let my stomach out." Passing the dreaded 50 marker, she expected that her days on camera were numbered. Watching CBS veteran Walter Cronkite age on air, Barbara used to predict with envious resignation, "He's beloved as Uncle Walter, but I'll never be Aunt Barbara." But her fears were not realized. At a party in the spring of 2005, I reminded Barbara that she had clocked in another quarter century at the top of her game. She laughed and allowed herself a little gloat: "Here I am, still on the air in my seventies! I think age is not an issue if you're liked."

From Pleasing to Mastery

The great transition in the passage to Second Adulthood for women is to move from pleasing to mastery. In our First Adulthood, we survive by figuring out how to please and perform for the powerful people who protect and reward us: parents, teachers, mates, and bosses. But by our midforties, we are all looking for greater mastery over our environment—emotional, physical, and vocational. It is in her fifties that a woman is fully ready to speak with her own voice. She might sound like one of my interviewees: "I've spent fifty years of my life pleasing everyone—my teachers, my bosses, my boyfriends, my husband, my children. Now," she said, "I care about pleasing *some* people and the rest can just go fly a kite!"

At 50, one stands on the mountaintop of the life span with a thrilling 360-degree view in all directions. The surge of potential power can be overwhelming. A sense of power in one's ability to influence events and control the way things turn out has been proven, in studies, to be a built-in self-fulfilling prophecy. Among the thousands of women I have interviewed about turning 50 in research for *New Passages* and for this book, I continue to find this mind-shift from pleasing to mastery to be nearly universal. More recently, the MacArthur Foundation studies on aging in America found that "people who increased their sense of mastery also increased their amount of productive activity." The study's authors, John Rowe, M.D., and Robert Kahn, Ph.D., found definitive proof that the shift to a greater belief in oneself *can be created* by midlifers. It takes three important elements to make the shift:

- First, the opportunity to take a specific action that challenges you (such as speaking in public for the first time)
- Second, support and reassurance from others (a mate, adult children, coach, friends)
- Third, the experience of succeeding at a new action and feedback from others that confirms your success

Even famous women, who one might assume were always confident and self-directed, undergo this shift. When Tina Brown looks back on the streak of career moves she made in her thirties and forties—from re-vamping *Vanity Fair* to running *The New Yorker* to creating her own magazine, *Talk,* while carrying two pregnancies, then mothering two little children and presiding over endless publicity parties with her equally high-profile husband—the whole saga leaves her breathless. A writer at heart, Tina had to let that passion go underground while she was a magazine executive. What she appreciates about getting older is suddenly finding that only *now* is she starting to feel liberated.

"While you're in that tunnel of work-kids-work-kids-work-kids, you can't imagine that your life will ever be different," she told me. "And at least for a mother, you're in that tunnel for a very long time. You think it might never end, and then no one will want you."

What she discovered coming out of the tunnel was quite the opposite. It is only since she turned 50, free of corporate restraints and merely tolerated by children now in their late teenage years, that she has been able to revive her dream: to be a writer. Tina also pulled off the amazing feat of creating her own TV show for the first time at the age of 50. Live on air, she looked completely at ease making smart, funny, spontaneous conversation, but this required mastery of a phobia she had always harbored about TV.

In an interview, Tina surprised me by admitting "I used to be very reserved when I was a young writer. When you're younger, you're far more inhibited by the need not to offend, but after fifty, the wit comes home to roost and you get much freer with it. I've noticed that women over fifty who've arrived somewhere are more confident about expressing their opinions. 'Why shouldn't I just say what I think?' "

Affluent women who can afford highlights, spa weeks, and expensive doctors have always been able to look better longer. But the real engine of extended vitality comes from within, says Tina. "I think it's more about self-assurance and the sense, today, that you have got another act. And it's happening all over."

When she held an eighteenth birthday party for her son, Tina invited a half-dozen of his teachers and tutors. "These were not high-profile media ladies. I remembered them as slightly dowdy women, but now they were all more stylishly dressed and they looked much younger than before." Two were seeking divorces. When Tina expressed her sympathies, they brushed off any pity. "This is something I've wanted for years," they told her. "And now I'm making it happen!"

Americans now *expect* to have a midlife crisis. By age 50, more than two thirds of baby-boomer women are reporting "a turbulent midlife transition," according to the massive study entitled "National Survey of Midlife Development in the United States," funded by the MacArthur Foundation. A further examination of that data found a dramatic turning point for women at 50. Only one quarter of women 35 to 49—fewer than in any other age group—said they had "fulfilled a special dream in the past five years." Surprisingly, this was the lowest ebb of fulfillment in their entire adult lives.

But for many women there is an upward turn around 50. The same data show that 36 percent of women between the ages of 50 and 64 report that they have reached some fulfilling goal or dream in the preceding five years (accomplishing something noteworthy; finding a partner; marriage; acquiring money or property). This suggests that more than one third of American females are well on their way to becoming seasoned women.

The picture for men is somewhat darker. The MacArthur data show that men's dream fulfillment goes downhill from their mid-thirties on, sinking to 28 percent of men between the ages of 50 and 64.

But there is time to change—and every reason to start making that shift *right now.* Soon, every sector of our consumer society will be wooing older boomers and making their lives easier. Why? They are riding a demographic tsunami.

The number of Americans over 65 will surpass the number of Americans under age 20—*in this decade.*

A "Little Death" and Rebirth

Psychologically, an old self has to die before a new self can be born, whether one recognizes it or not. The striving and competing that lend a furious intensity to our First Adulthood are now likely to feel more like a narrow and futile chase after the illusion of ultimate success. Men and women who pour most of their energy into their careers begin to complain about the dull repetition of duties and ask: *Why do I have to work so hard? Where is the meaning?* The search for meaning in whatever we do becomes a universal preoccupation of our Second Adulthood. I've called it the Meaning Crisis.

After healthy, educated, emancipated women come out the other end of the midlife passage, they can look forward to greater freedom to make choices than at any other time in their lives. Almost anything is possible—creative rebirths, business start-ups, educational refinishing, a plunge into politics, bailing out of a bad marriage, new permission for flirtation, fun, and second-chance romances, or the evolution of a truly seasoned marriage that combines mature sexual pleasure and a soul connection.

The increased life span alone, of course, does not promise a rich Second Adulthood. The added years are merely a blank slate; it's what we write on them that makes the difference.

Locating Your Age and Stage

Before we can appreciate what is involved in reaching for a higher state of love, sex, spirituality, and passion in Second Adulthood, we need to have in mind the developmental tasks that are linked to our chronological age as we move along the adult life cycle.

Each new stage, as I see it, is signaled by a sense of disequilibrium and uncertainty. We enter a passage—a transition during which we have a heightened potential for healthy change and a heightened danger of doing something destructive to avoid change. During these passages, previous choices are questioned, signaling the onset of a new stage and the necessity to alter or replace our goals with ones more appropriate to the new stage. A redefined and extended ladder of the stages of the Second Adulthood (originally laid out in *New Passages*) appears on the following pages. Locating yourself on this ladder will better prepare you to move on to new possibilities.

Predictable Passages of Second Adulthood

Pits to Peak Passage

A period of gathering disequilibrium in the mid- to late forties shakes up the more stable stage that precedes it. Women and men are simultaneously undergoing the dying of youth and stumbling into the infancy of their Second Adulthood.

As women begin to notice signs of aging, there is a Vanity Crisis. Women in their mid-forties often feel they are sliding into a pit, darkened by the shadow of menopause up ahead. Except for late-baby mothers, this is also the usual time when children begin leaving the nest. There is a natural mourning for the loss of fertility, which can precipitate a commonplace terror: *What if overnight I turn into Old Woman?*

But at 50, as documented by my research and many other studies, women commonly feel they are just beginning to reach their peak.

Feisty Fifties

Older is bolder, and today's women in their fifties are more feisty than fearful. They don't necessarily want a man or a role to define them anymore. They are defining themselves.

Our narcissistic need to believe we are still young is challenged by the men on the street to whom we become invisible. That is the signal to intensify our other attractions: wit and wisdom, energy and enthusiasm, unexploited skills and talents, and the capacity to enliven others' dreams, provided we develop one of our own. As women in their fifties develop greater mastery over their emotions and their environment, they expand their control and gain deepened confidence, power, and inner harmony.

The mortality issue is unavoidable at this stage, if it hasn't intruded earlier. Odds are that around these years a parent, a contemporary, a mate, or we ourselves will have a life accident, one of those events we can neither predict nor prevent—a health crisis such as breast cancer or a husband's prostate cancer; the unexpected death of a family member, friend, or colleague; a catastrophic career setback; or a war that may put an adult child in harm's way. Any such life accident can pitch us into fear or depression, but, more positively, it can precipitate the Meaning Crisis. The acknowledgment of death can be an enormous asset in one's life; it pushes us to search for meaningfulness.

The search for meaning, in whatever we do, becomes the universal preoccupation of the Second Adulthood. It is based on a spiritual imperative: even as we strive for individual authenticity, we also yearn to believe in and belong to some reality larger than the self.

As women age, we become more focused, more managerial, more aggressive, more political, and very often feel that "At last, it's time for me. It's time for my contribution to the world."

Passage to the Age of Mastery

The middle years, between 50 and 65, constitute the apex of adult life—the Age of Mastery. For women, the passage to be made is from pleasing to mastery. Most women come to realize they have been defined in their First Adulthood by their relation to others—the parents, husbands, children, bosses, and mentors for whom they performed. Now is the time to construct one's own new Second Adulthood identity.

Psychologically, something has to die before a new self can be born. The "little death" of the idealized dream of the First Adulthood precipitates something of a mourning phase before we can emerge from the passage and say, "Okay, now I have a new life; there is a new part of me that is allowed to grow."

Selective Sixties

For the vast majority of American and European women and men today, the sixties are a stage where a maximum freedom of choice coexists with a minimum of physical limitations. Your mind is still working, your body is still working, and you have the benefit of a mature perspective on life—the first time you possess that combination. The opportunities offered for expanding the meaning of your life are unlimited, but you have to choose selectively and focus your energies. Nobody can dictate to you anymore, nor can you avoid taking responsibility for your own life.

There is a new freedom for playfulness. At this stage you have permission to select out those people and things that are truly important to you and to say no to others.

With retirement, there is a heightened potential for making another leap of growth but also the danger of lapsing into entropy or depression. Late-life learning is a new possibility and a priority for those who want to remain vigorous of mind. Paid work, perhaps part-time, is valued more highly than unpaid, but selecting the most meaningful voluntary activities can keep you engaged, and engagement is essential to successful aging.

Passage to the Age of Unity

The years of late Second Adulthood, from 65 to 85 or beyond, provide the chance for wholeness, as opposed to the dividedness of so much of earlier life. The goal is a coalescence of all that has been lived and learned into a sense of unity in our values and purposes. Contentment comes from what Emerson called "the sacredness of private integrity."

Life's opportunities expand in proportion to our courage to seek them out. If we are still growing, not retreating into self-pity or depression, the heart expands, love finds many avenues, and we enjoy being loved for who we have become as people. This can be a period of grace and generosity. Erik Erikson, the father of adult development theory, described the primary task of this seventh stage of adult development as "generativity"—the voluntary obligation to care for and about others.

Spontaneous Seventies

These years beyond getting and spending and status seeking offer the chance to become a "pilgrim of the soul," as Yeats phrased it. The ultimate task of self-mastery is to develop an appreciation for the complexity of life, to be able to control first impulses and resist taking sides in conflict, to be a wise mediator in the paradoxes of life. For those who are able to view the world with bemused detachment, this allows greater spontaneity and gaiety.

But life from here on also becomes an endurance event. A clear choice must be made to continue to grow, intellectually and spiritually, and to counter the drift toward passivity with disciplined daily physical activity. Otherwise, the body will gradually decay. The most current studies of successful aging reveal that *daily* exercise, both physical and mental, and nurturing engagement with others must become a commitment that begins *before* the seventies.

Passage to Cultivation or Isolation

Erikson conceived of the eighth and final stage of adult development as a struggle between integrity and despair. Integrity, he suggested, is a state of mind assured of order and meaning, a capacity for postnarcissistic love, and the serenity to bless and defend one's own life history.

I have modified this passage to emphasize the importance of "cultivation," borrowing the agricultural term for refreshing the soil to improve its condition. In human terms, there are many ways to turn over the soil in which we can continue to grow, to fertilize ourselves with new friends and activities, and to weed out the habits or negative people who might choke off our perennial blooms.

This is also the stage of the guru. We have the choice of cultivating younger "students" of life and passing on our knowledge or gradually slipping into isolation as friends die off and are not replaced. Engagement in community activities is vital to prolonging social contacts and perpetuating the sense of mastery.

Being a grandparent is one of the most valued and treasured roles that we can perform from the seventies onward. We bring to the table not only toys and surprises, easy laughter and unqualified love; we become the polestars that will guide our progeny long after we have departed.

Enduring Eighties, Noble Nineties, and the Ascent to Centenarian

People who enjoy strong connections with others live longer. Widows who maintain friendships with others, and who reach out to form new relationships in later life, are healthier in mind and body. It is also a fact that the vast majority of centenarians retain close ties to their families.

Courage and stoicism in the face of inevitable assaults on the body and the aftereffects of medical treatment seem to fortify inner strength. To be among the successfully long-lived, we must have cultivated some specific purpose or joy to wake up for, a reason to fight another day, an appetite for seeing another sunset.

The ultimate opportunity is to cultivate "second sight," an awakening to a broader view of past and future and possibly life after death. We call this state of mind transcendence. The Japanese call it *satori.* Buddhists speak of becoming a Bodhisattva, one who has reached Enlightenment but postpones Nirvana in order to teach others how to reach Enlightenment.

One major goal of this book is to open a window on the full second half of the female life cycle, which rarely is depicted in popular entertainment as it is actually lived today. Although I interviewed many men in my research for this book, it was not possible to encompass the variations on the Second Adulthood for both sexes within one book. I hope to address men's pursuit of the passionate life in a future book.

A second objective is to show the many fresh and exciting new ways in which seasoned women are coupling and partnering, within and without marriage. In my latest research, I have found that the Sexual Diamond (the crossover of male/female characteristics in middle and later age) holds out even greater promise for new kinds of egalitarian partnerships in the mature stages of life. How do men and women respond to this new deal? Are we as evolved as we think we are?

My third and most important goal is to persuade you that it is worthwhile to pursue a more passionate life, despite the false starts, fears of rejection or ridicule, and inevitable disappointments.

Warning: I can't give you nice, neatly tied up success stories of women who jumped off the well-beaten path at 50 and found eternal bliss with their 25-year-old fitness instructors; nor can I give you stories of resurgent midlife marriages with five easy steps to an overnight transformation. The stories in this book are meant to give you the courage and inspiration to pursue your own path to the more passionate life. You will meet women whose new dreams are evolving nicely. You will learn about the insults some have weathered in breaking out of the stereotypes of the invisible, sexless older woman. You will also watch some take great leaps and stumble or fall hard, though most pick themselves up and feel they have learned something valuable. Their stories are not finished, and neither are they. Most of the women and men in this book are moving on, changing, growing, and living more passionately than ever.

Chapter 3

Tracking the Seasoned Woman

began my formal research by posting a simple questionnaire on my website. I illustrated it with a nineteenth-century painting by Gustave Courbet of a voluptuous woman reclining, naked, in a glen, and holding a parrot on her finger. The picture was doctored to make her hair silver-gray. The headline read, *"Sex for Women Over 50 Is for the Birds, Right?"* The idea was to mock the stereotype held pretty much around the world—that for women of menopausal age, sexual desire shuts down.*

It struck a chord.

Many of my respondents said they had been surprised to feel the exact opposite—a powerful resurgence of desire. And they aren't just fantasizing about sex and romance; many describe feeling an expansion of sexual freedom. They are not as willing as they once were to put up with the "stability" of a marriage devoid of real intimacy. And those who are single, unrestrained by the old "shoulds," are finding a new boldness to experiment. So many women now in midlife have a lot of catching up to do!

Another important research avenue was opened with the help of

---

* You will find the questionnaire in the Appendix. If you'd like to join the Seasoned Women's Network, where women over 45 talk about what we *really think,* log on to my website, www.gailsheehy.com, give your e-mail address, and you will be included in our ongoing conversation. You can fill out the questionnaire there and participate in my ongoing research.

ThirdAge, an online media and marketing website with more than a million and a half members, which focuses on the needs of midlife adults. I was asked to write articles about my ideas and theories on this stage of life and, in exchange, I could query its vast membership on their views of love, sex, dating, and passion over 50. A wealth of messages was posted, coming from every corner of the country and across the spectrum of reactions, from active seekers of sexual and spiritual connections, to married women who said they were "passionately enjoying sex with a lover" (sometimes referring to their husbands, sometimes not), to midlife singles too shy to try dating, to those who were unhappily married. Many postings led to one-on-one interviews and often a research trip to meet the women in person.

In the fall of 2003, I began asking my contacts around the country if they would set up group interviews with women 50 and over about romance, sex, and love. The response was immediate.

"OhmyGod, I'd love to be able to compare notes with other women my age!"

"My sister is divorced and having incredible sex with a young buck, and I'm married and jealous!"

"Can I join, even if I'm married?"

It was a telling question, but of course she could. Romance and long-term marriage are not mutually exclusive. I am using the concept of sex in a very expansive sense. Not infrequently, what remains of a love affair after the passionate attraction fades is a bond of warmth and affection that may grow into a nurturing relationship without sex. And those relationships, as you will read, sometimes evolve into the deepest of soul connections.

This is my fifteenth book, and I have never had such an easy time finding people who wanted to talk—despite the fact that it involved such private matters. I couldn't stop them! Women in this life stage are hungry for a safe setting in which to talk openly about finding their self-identities, about the delights and disasters of "dating" (a word many hate), their yearnings within marriage, or their passionate love affairs on the secret outskirts. They love sharing stories of their trepidations and exultations in new sexual encounters, about rekindled romances from their youth, about commuting relationships, rescued marriages, heartaches, and renewed hopes.

While this was not an academically stringent survey, the results were nevertheless provocative. One might have expected the preponderance of replies to reflect the frustration and loneliness of *Desperate Housewives,* or, worse, to echo the bitter divorcées of *The First Wives Club.* Surprise! My subjects naturally divided into five groups: Passionates; Seekers; WMDs (Women Married, Dammit!); SQs (Status Quos); and LLs (Lowered Libidos). By far the largest group of respondents can be classified as "Passionates."

Passionates (40% of Total)

These are healthy, independent, sexy women anywhere between their late forties and eighties, usually working and able to take care of themselves financially. They are passionate about their work or a cause, or in pursuit of a new dream or spiritual quest.

Half of the Passionates are divorced and over 50. They seldom have dating problems, enjoy a lot of sexual activity, and are most likely to be involved with someone romantically but not eager to remarry, at least for now. Most of them find that a new lover is a wonderful antidote to menopause.

Married and cohabiting Passionates are often reveling in a remarriage made in midlife or a new lover. Many others have long-standing marriages to mates they cherish and with whom they enjoy making love. They often say they are enjoying a resurgence of romance since the children left or have introduced novelty into their habitual sexplay.

Widowed Passionates are among the most hopeful. Most of them have enjoyed marriage. They know how to share their lives, miss the camaraderie of marriage, and eagerly anticipate being able to find another mate.

Only a handful of the Passionates have never been married.

Here are some typical experiences related to me by the Passionates:

"I'm over fifty and proud of it," Rachel offered even before I asked her age. A classic divorced Passionate, she had endured a sexually mori-bund marriage for more years than she likes to recall. Her husband found another love, and for the first year of her separation, she says, she felt burned, depressed, uninterested in sex. A management consultant, she said, "You go into different offices still carrying an inner image of yourself as somewhere in your thirties. Suddenly, you find that all the other people in the office *are* in their thirties, and *you're not*—you're even older than the boss!"

When friends began pushing blind dates on her, she turned in self-defense to the Internet. "To be honest, my number one motivation was to prove I was still attractive," she admitted. "I also had a lot of pent-up sexual energy, and the taste of freedom was exhilarating."

In more than two years of active posting on Internet dating sites, Rachel has met more than a hundred men. She describes many of her ear-lier dates as "nerds, socially isolated men who aren't high achievers, and boring!" She continues to be surprised at the many men in their twenties who reply to her posts. "They profess to like older women, and some have a pretty good rap. I guess they're looking to get laid, and they have a fan-tasy that I'm Teri Hatcher"—the screwball Susan on *Desperate House-wives* who is locked out of her house, nude. Rachel is too pragmatic to rule out exchanging e-mails with married men, more of whom she finds are "quality men" and with whom she has developed some interest-ing platonic friendships. She has more recently enjoyed dating a George-town professor, a medical center attorney, and a bicoastal strategist. All of this experience made her more strategic at "fishing" in the vast seas of Internet dating sites and pulling out a catch she might want to keep.

Sexual chemistry finally struck when she met a cerebral type who works in a think tank and said he likes to be involved with women "in their goddess years." He is typical of men who have mastered Internet dating: they develop skills that give them a competitive advantage. This academic didn't have a big bank account or look like Harrison Ford, but he'd made himself a champion at tantric sex. "Your pleasure is my plea-sure" was his signature line. He taught her how to delay her response and enjoy multiple orgasms.

"My sex life is richer now than ever," Rachel says. "This man can arouse me from across a crowded room. To know not only what pleases me, but to be able to ask for it, and *get it,* is astonishing to me—and I'm now fifty-five!"

*   *   *

Kaylie, a divorcée who remarried in her fifties, was frank but thankful for what she has: "Even though my libido is lower since menopause—I don't think about sex as much—my new husband [of five years] makes love to me with a leisurely pace and my orgasms are the most powerful I have ever had. I appreciate my husband's body more than I ever appreciated a man's body before. I have been married twice before and lived by myself for the better part of my forties. Likely a good part of my attitude is the result of going through the mid-forties passage you described in *New Passages.*"

*   *   *

Rita Mae offers another illustration of the optimistic outlook of the Passionates: "I'm turning fifty-four soon and have always loved sex— just not with my husband. He was a good lover, but abusive in many ways, and after years of living with that, my love died. We have been living apart for two years now, and I've been in an intimate relationship with a man older than I am. We connected the first time we talked, and the sex has been fantastic! I never thought this would happen to me, but the holding and kissing and just lying next to that special man and feeling our skin touching is such a wonderful experience—I *need that!*"

*   *   *

A widowed Passionate, Patricia from Arkansas, announced in her e-mail, "I was reintroduced to my sexuality in midlife, and, indeed, to life itself!" In a follow-up interview, it was apparent that she is enjoying the sense of mastery from having come through a dark passage.

Patricia was dealt a bad hand when she married a much older man whose heart failed shortly thereafter. Their sexual connection withered. She remained faithful to him for the next eighteen years, until he died of a stroke. No sinking into the aspic of self-pity for this widow. She tried

Date.com, eHarmony, and Great Expectations. "All helped me 'get my groove back,' " she says. "Now, at fifty-six, I feel the confidence and freedom to be *me* like never before. I have a very healthy, romantic, and actively sexual relationship with a slightly older man. We've each had rough spots in our lives. We respect the courage it took for each of us to go on, as much as we respect what we have together now, trusting that each of us can continue to grow and reach beyond."

These typical experiences of Passionates over 50 are living proof of a scientific fact shown by many studies: when all the parameters of sexuality are compared, the number one factor in enhancing sexual desire and response among women is a new partner.*

Seekers (20% of Total)

These are healthy, single women who indicate they are "hungry for sex" or will "never give up" and who are actively seeking companions or sexual partners but are not yet having much luck. Some are so new to the role of Seeker, they're not sure how to play it. Many others describe themselves as "frustrated" or "disappointed with men and society," feel the cards are stacked against them, and believe that most men over 50 are aiming for younger partners. Seekers, too, like the Passionates, are usually working and able to take care of themselves financially. Most have not yet found a new passion, and many are still nursing old grudges from previous relationships. Their expectations tend to be unrealistic, at least at this point.

Many of the Seekers say that changes in their desire or response with menopause came as a surprise. They report that they are using vaginal estrogen, hormones, or self-stimulation to combat the changes. Despite their frustration, they are continu-

* The largest study—of 438 women—is the Melbourne Women's Study by Lorraine Dennerstein, reported in 2005 at the University of Melbourne: "The Relative Effects of Hormones and Relationship Factors on Sexual Functioning of Women through the Natural Menopausal Transition."

ing to seek, which distinguishes them from the Status Quos and Lowered Libidos.

Widowed Seekers often say they miss the camaraderie of married life, and some are looking for new husbands rather than just dates.

Typical of replies from the Seekers was one from Andrea, a former probation officer whose passion was to pick up the dream of her twenties. She wanted to be a practicing poet—after all, as an undergraduate, she had been a *published* poet.

When she had her first child at 40, her priorities changed. She retired from court work to develop a private psychotherapy practice and have more time to enjoy motherhood. While her practice grew into a viable one, her marriage deteriorated. She was in her late fifties, with an adolescent son, when she realized that the time had come to file for divorce. An even greater rupture followed when, not long after, her only child went off to college.

Now, at last, there was time to seek her dream. She was determined to find the metro poetry community where she lived. Over the course of a year or two, she became a part of the local poetry network and made new friends. She was asked to give readings and is now published in more than twenty poetry journals.

Hard as it is to find suitable single men in the Midwest, she says, Andrea met a distinguished older retired attorney. She was still good-looking, in the final blaze of youth. The age difference did not bother her; it even crossed her mind that dating a gentleman of 73 would make her feel younger. It didn't. His energy level was half of hers. Although he complimented her and offered rather chaste goodnight kisses, he refused her offers to stop for coffee. His frequent references to sex were only ironic. She surmised that he might be impotent. After some months, she stopped dating him.

Being new at the game, Andrea says she finds dating and sex in one's fifties as baffling as traveling in a foreign country where one doesn't know the language: "I'm not always entirely sure of appropriate boundaries—

how much to ask, how much to tell. I plan to work and write more. I volunteer. I still feel young in every respect. I'm hoping for a mate, but not necessarily to marry. I really desire reciprocal love. I'm feeling sexually passionate."

In spite of a full social and professional life, there are times, she says, especially in the depths of the midwestern winter when her son is away, that she feels intensely lonely. "I hate the thought of sort of shriveling up and don't expect I will. This 'story' is probably a fairly generic illustration of women my age. I don't regret divorcing—even at such a late age, fifty-seven—but I did not think I'd experience the loneliness I sometimes do feel. We need success stories and encouragement."

Is it possible to find love after you've been alone and sexless for years? Let me share with you one of the many success stories I have collected.

She Met Him at the Mall

After Susan's second divorce at the age of 43, she went through a long dry period—what she calls "my busy period." She decided she didn't want to date—"Been there, done that"—and became consumed with building her own design business. Her friends kept wanting to fix her up; she told them she had no time for that.

Last year Susan surprised her best girlfriend by saying, "I think I'd like to let a man into my life now."

Where did that shift come from? I asked Susan.

"I'd just turned sixty. I think it came from my deciding that my career was only going to last X number of years, and then what? I don't want to work all my life. I want to travel, read, lecture, teach classes. Then I realized I'm not sharing my life with anyone. I was busying myself—I always had an agenda, so nothing spontaneous could happen.

"So I just let go."

Susan scaled her business way back, let her employees go, and closed down her warehouse. Within months, it happened. Susan was in the mall on Christmas Eve. She spotted a very tall, handsome, impeccably dressed gentleman leaning against the wall and talking on a cell phone. The sight amused her. Susan herself is a pocket-size size six and platinum blond. She smiled at the gentleman, a signaling sort of smile, and kept walking. She passed another store, stopped, turned around, ran into him again, and gave him another smile. He followed her into the next store and walked right up to speak to her.

"I'm old enough to know if I don't follow my instincts, we'll never pass this way again," he said, "so would you have coffee with me after the holidays?" He was very well spoken and younger, but not all that much younger, she guessed. In the past, she would have replied, "Gee, thanks very much, but I think not." Instead, she said, "Yes."

Susan ricocheted between a laissez-faire attitude—"I don't need a man in my life"—to feeling possessive and insecure about capturing this man.

"It is just opening the door," she now says. "Even after a decade-long dry period, a mind-shift can result in behavior shift. Once I was more open, I must have sent out that signal."

Susan and her new man have now been together for seventeen months. She still doesn't know how old he is, and he inquired about her age only once. She gave him double-talk. He called back and said he didn't care.

"WMDs" (Women Married, Dammit!)
(15% of Total)

These are women who are frustrated by marriages that have been emotionally dead and sexually moribund for some time, or who feel victimized by a mate who is a chronic drinker, adulterer, or poor provider, etc. But for utilitarian reasons, they are not ready or able to initiate change. And they don't have a new passion or spiritual direction.

The greatest proportion of WMDs have given up on sex. They are turned off or angry and say they are "too busy to be bothered by any of this," or they have different interests now. Typical of responses in this category is a woman of 60 who writes, "I'm bored and resent being the purse. I want to be in a relationship that is reciprocal."

> About one third of the WMDs are having, or have had, af-
> fairs. Some are hungry for sex, but either they, or their mates, no
> longer find each other desirable partners. This falloff can hap-
> pen with partners who are older or younger.

The e-mails from WMDs sound like this:

"I'm still as interested in sex as ever, but my husband, who is only one year older, has lost all interest because of his physical problems and being depressed."

"I married a man 10 years younger, just a year ago, and now we have no sex at all. He says he has 'issues' from the past and no desire."

"I've been married 28 years and never realized the price. I wish I didn't love men so much, otherwise I'd probably just be with women. Am I a bit bitter? Yes."

The WMDs are even more frustrated when they hear from their divorced or widowed friends about a romantic and sexual playing field out there that sounds too good to be true. And maybe it is: the grass always looks greener on the other side. Many WMDs say they wish they could go back to dating but can't because they're married. Others say, "It might be better out there, but I can't imagine anything worse than dating again." Or "I've taken care of one man all these years; I couldn't begin to find the energy or desire to take care of another one." Their frustrations are revealing: "If I were single, I would love a relationship with someone with separate homes and bank accounts, but who'd be a great regular playmate and sexual partner."

A small proportion of the WMDs are more hopeful. Marilou, a traditional southern woman, thought when she separated from her husband five years ago that she had lost interest in having a real relationship and good sex. "I thought my children were all I needed for the rest of my life," she wrote. "Then I reunited with an old boyfriend from high school and discovered that passion was still inside me. To feel like a girl again, to cry, to long for love, they were all inside me, dormant." Having found out that she is still alive as a woman, Marilou is hopeful about creating a deeper relationship with her old high school sweetheart.

"SQs" *(Status Quos)* *(12% of Total)*

These women are not necessarily unhappy, just resigned. They don't have a new dream or a new love. At this point, they feel the status quo is preferable to the risk and discomfort of change.

Many SQs have long-standing marriages in which sex is only a memory. They don't seem to care as long as they are able to preserve the social structure of marriage and enjoy strong bonds with their adult children and grandchildren. Sometimes, their husbands are off having sex with someone else, probably younger and thinner, to which the SQs turn a blind eye.

SQs who are divorced or widowed say they are "wishful but too shy" to consider dating over 50 or "clueless" about how to seek out companions. Others are "hungry for sex" but think they're too old. Some are simply resigned to living out their days without a partner. They may be fully engaged in their professional lives, very active in their community, or taking care of a frail parent. Some SQs express hope that the "right person" may come along, but put no effort into the search, vastly decreasing the likelihood that their status will change.

Choosing to be an SQ is a more positive decision than lapsing into being a WMD, whose passive anger may be toxic to herself and those around her. Many women opt for the status quo in their First Adulthood to maintain a stable home for their children and keep hoping things will improve, but if the nest empties and the marriage, too, remains empty, the SQ becomes resigned.

Other SQs are long divorced. One of my website respondents in her late fifties describes herself as "pretty" and "without problems in attracting men" but admits she retreats from them. "I just look at them as a 'heartache' waiting to happen. I miss the love factor in my life. But the awful, intense, hurtful feelings of a breakup are too much for me to bear, so I go on my merry way alone."

In withdrawing from sex and intimate relationships, SQs may have more energy and passion to devote to other pursuits or good works. A website responder who identifies herself as a loner said she is revolted by the idea of dating over 50: "I'm 54, and I found a passion better than men (at least at this point). I went skydiving and loved it. It's a more expensive passion, but much cheaper than a relationship or a marriage. I can come and go as I please and spend all night surfing the Web for skydiving gear, and not have to answer to anyone. In my last relationship—with a kid 13 years younger than me—I learned my bullshit meter is out of whack. So best to stay in the clouds. 'Cause I can."

The small percentage of SQs who have never married indicate that they have well-formed lives and are unwilling to "sacrifice" for a relationship.

Another website response summed up the sad and self-defeating reasons some older SQs may give up on passion of any kind. A woman of 70 who is divorced and not interested in sex cited the big three: "Too old. Too fat. Too scared."

LLs (Lowered Libidos) (12% of Total)

These are women who have totally given up on sex or who "grin and bear it." Most are married, most of the rest are divorced, and a very few have never married, but all indicate they have experienced lowered libido since menopause. The saddest fact about this group is their admission that they are doing nothing about it—they don't take hormones or use vaginal estrogen and rarely even use self-stimulation or try to introduce novelty into their marriages.

Some of the divorced LLs say they would like to negotiate a limited, nonsexual "couple" relationship for the purpose of social events and traveling but do not really make an effort. (Some of the Passionates and Seekers are also looking for a nonsexual relationship, but they put much more effort into its pursuit.)

These categories are not fixed pigeonholes. They are fluid; any one of us might occupy any given pigeonhole at different points. Just about any woman might be classified a "WMD" from time to time, wondering what she is missing by sticking with a less-than-perfect marriage. Of course, all marriages are less than perfect, some just more "less" than others. And we probably all feel like SQs in some periods, when we're just treading water or trying to survive. Many of the Seekers were SQs for years until something lit their fire in midlife—even rather late in midlife. For example:

"The person I was when I left my marriage, after thirty-nine years, and the person I am now, are two different people," says Dani, a southern California woman who enjoyed being a mother and who worked on commission at a job that gave her little joy. "My husband was my passionate love, but I don't think I ever was his," she can now admit with equanimity. "I needed more affection, but I stuck with the status quo, and I'm not sorry. I wasn't ready." Like many boomer women, Dani had grown up between divorced parents who constantly tore each other down, which tore her in two. She didn't want to become bitter like her mother. Many years of her married life were happy and fun, but at some indefinable point she crossed into that haze of habitual motion that one recognizes only in retrospect as just walking through. She contented herself, as do many married SQs, by saying, "At least I have a life."

The arc of her passage from a passive SQ to an active Seeker is familiar: "One day I looked over at him in bed—this man I'd loved as a teenager—and I thought, 'It's gone.' I had just shut down." Her children had left home. She hated her work. Her husband had had a heart attack and was clutching at life in every direction but hers—using Viagra but probably cheating, consumed with his new passion for boating with his guy friends, and telling her he wasn't sure he loved her or wanted to be married anymore.

"I kept saying, 'I've got one foot out the door, but I'll never be able to leave this man.' " Two months before her sixtieth birthday, Dani closed the door behind her.

She had already begun a pilgrimage of the soul that prepared the ground for her passage. "I'm Jewish but not real religious," she says. While searching for a new dream, she offered to volunteer at a life-coaching center for women in midlife. "I learned to remember to breathe," she says, a first step away from sleepwalking through life. Dani collected big fat Buddhas and rubbed their bellies to remind herself to breathe and smile.

And there had already been a spark.

"OhmyGod, Jimmy just e-mailed me!" she had shouted from her computer. She ran through the house looking for her husband and visiting children to tell them all about Jimmy—her first love, at summer camp, in the swoon of pubescent sexual heat. She hadn't seen him in forty-five years, but after a few months of exchanging exhilarating e-mails, Dani knew: "If I see this man in person, I'll sleep with him." That gave her the final push to walk out the door.

Dani's story crystallizes one of the unique appeals of rekindling an old flame. "This man knows more about me than anybody on the face of the earth, and I know more about him. And we were best friends first. That gives me more comfort than my husband of so many years." Jimmy told her again and again that she was beautiful, an affirmation that every woman longs for, especially in the middle years, when she fears she is molting into Old Woman. Dani noted that Jimmy was short and stocky and, by any objective standard, not nearly as fit as her husband. "But all he has to do is touch my arm and I'm aroused."

With her husband, Dani could never talk about sex. They made love in bed with the lights out, period. But with her old camp beau, she can talk about what her needs are. "This man only wants to please me, and I want to please him," she says. "I couldn't do the same things with my husband, because we'd built up patterns over the years; we'd have been embarrassed to suggest it."

What would come of this affair? Dani's old camp boyfriend was married, and his life was on the opposite coast. But he had made her realize that there was life after her marriage. She consulted a therapist, who taught her to remember what flight attendants always say: "Put your own oxygen mask on first"—another reminder to breathe. When she finally got up the courage to tell her husband, she said, "I've spent too many years living your life, I can't do this anymore." He was shocked. But it didn't take Dani long after moving out to find herself.

"I remember the exact day," she says with a broad smile in her voice. "I went to a wedding in Napa Valley with friends and stayed by myself in a little B and B. The next morning I walked into town and got a latte, the sun was shining, the grapes were bursting on the vines, and I sang out, 'Hot damn, I found a new best friend—me.' "

Since then, Dani says she has never felt as lonely as she did living with her husband. And the act of leaving him has prompted him to show more emotional warmth toward their children and grandchildren. She and her ex-husband are now friends who can go out to dinner with the grandkids once a week and often share holidays and even movies. One of her daughters told her, "Mom, I'm so proud of you, you should have done this years ago."

Dani has not yet become an active Seeker, but she is on the path. "I'm just getting up the nerve, but I'm ready and willing," she says. "I do love sex, and I never thought I could be this passionate—at the age of sixty-two!"

✦   ✦   ✦

Women gathered with me in groups from coast to coast: East Coast suburban wives and divorced professional women in Stamford, Connecticut, and Red Bank, New Jersey; therapists who had started a singles' group on the North Shore of Long Island. In the southern states I met with minimum-wage women in eastern Arkansas; affluent women in Fort Worth, Texas; and a clique of divorced and dating nurses in Tulsa, Oklahoma. I talked with academic and corporate women in Minneapolis, Minnesota, and sex counselors in Las Vegas, Nevada. In Santa Fe, New Mexico, I gathered with a dozen artists and political activists, and a separate group of lesbian women. In California, there were three groups. In Berkeley, active users of the online dating service Match.com compared experiences with clients of a traditional matchmaking service, CheckMates; in a San Francisco beauty salon, an informal network of unmarried women from age 50 to nearly 90 gathered; and in southern California's Orange County, I met with members of a new women's network called WomanSage. In Scottsdale, Arizona, I talked to men and women members of an active senior center who love to dance.

There were also three men's groups: a network of early forced retirees now working from home in Queens, New York; a group of divorced professional men from Manhattan and Connecticut; and a group of men in the San Francisco Bay area whose wives had walked out on them once the children were grown. In these lively storytelling sessions, two of the enduring myths about older women were exploded: one, that women aren't interested in sex after menopause; and two, that there are no available men out there who aren't losers or chasing younger women. One former globe-trotting wire service reporter in his late fifties, who keeps his body rock solid by biking around New York, spoke to this when I asked him to spell out the comparative advantages of dating a woman over 50 and a woman twenty years younger.

"The woman over fifty will go out with me," he deadpanned.

Hearing so many fascinating anecdotes in our group discussions, I went back to many of the women and men to do lengthy follow-up interviews. When deeper questions were raised by my participants' experiences, I discussed them with some of the most seasoned professionals in pertinent fields: psychologists and psychiatrists, sociologists, anthropologists, gynecologists, sex therapists, physicians who specialize in male and female sexual dysfunction, and the dogged researchers at the U.S. Census Bureau, the MacArthur Foundation, AARP, Unmarried America (formerly the membership division of the American Association for Single People), the National Marriage Project at Rutgers University, the New England Centenarian Study at Boston University, and others.

◆   ◆   ◆

Sadly, some people find the subject of older women and sex repugnant, or perhaps threatening. My own young editorial assistants turned up their noses when asked to transcribe the first interviews I did with women over 50 about their sex, love, and dating habits: "Eeeyou." But at the end of the day, they came to me with expressions of amazement and relief. "Thank God—there's life after we get older!" said Miranda McLeod, a dazzling 23-year-old. "We're all taught to believe that our twenties are the best years of our lives—we're at our peak, physically, sexually, and socially—and that's tragic, to think this is as good as it gets. Reading these interviews, you realize you've been fed a lie. It's arbitrary to say that the twenties are the peak of anything. These women keep saying at fifty and over they're having the best sex of their lives—it's so great to have something to look forward to!"

And unlike earlier generations of adult daughters who were likely to be scandalized and censorious of older single mothers who became romantically active again, many contemporary daughters are cheering on their single moms. Catherine Sweeney, another of my able editorial assistants, gets frequent phone calls from her divorced mother to discuss dating protocols. "Of course you should accept his offer to go to Thailand for a week," Catherine will say, "and don't bother booking a separate hotel room." Her mom called from the plane. "I could never do this without your support."

With all the vicissitudes of middle and later life, seasoned women have a great luxury—free time—that young working women striving for credentials in their twenties and sleep-deprived working moms in their thirties and forties can only dream about. The children of seasoned women are grown, and if not gone, they can at least pick up their own clothes and amuse themselves. The women are likely to be senior enough in their work to have some discretion over their schedule, or, increasingly likely, they work for themselves and very likely from home. They have time to go to the gym, time to hop on the back of a Harley or a raft down the Colorado or run off on a romantic escapade to Paris should the offer arise—whether doing it within a reinvigorated marriage or with a guy met on Match.com.

This book is not about celebrities. It is about real people, some of whom asked for pseudonyms, but many of whom were proud to allow the use of their own names. Their stories will show myriad ways in which the passionate life is sought, who succeeds, and the pitfalls to avoid. Parts II through VI of the book will elucidate the phases of the pursuit and how it works in the lives of women from the age of 45 all the way to 100. The case histories are based on personal interviews with more than two hundred women and a smaller number of men.

Most belong to the middle class and some are upper middle class. But among my respondents, class level does not appear to be a significant factor in determining whether a woman is a Passionate or a Seeker or a WMD. The Passionates range from a Florida woman of 52 living with a younger lover who drives a Ford, works full-time, and takes inexpensive vacations, to a California widow of 57 who dates, drives a Lexus, manages her investments, and vacations in Europe.

Among the Seekers are some who are not economically independent or in robust health. Gladys, a 51-year-old midwestern woman who is married and drives a minivan, wishes desperately that she could live on her own.

"I would be happily divorced and maybe in a more meaningful relationship," she says. "It probably sounds cold, but I stay with my husband because of what he provides. There must be many women like me in our generation." Gladys had a kidney transplant in her forties. She worked all the while she was on dialysis and came home to teenagers and a husband who complained that she was running up too many bills. "The job kept me sane," she says, to explain why she stayed with a job that gave her no health benefits. When her youngest graduated from high school, she decided to be free—"Well, as free as I could be without upsetting them all." She indulged herself in a relationship with a younger man. "I don't know if you could call it a love affair, but he made me feel good about myself again, and we both love to dance!" She continues to seek out friendships with other men for fun and companionship, "nothing serious." With the schools cutting their budgets, she expects she will probably lose her job soon, but her outlook is hopeful. "Now that I'm fifty-one, going back to school doesn't seem like anything I'd like to do—but who knows!"

The WMDs include a retired flight attendant who wishes she had a livelier companion than her husband to share all her free flight miles. Another WMD would love to divorce but must fight to keep her home so she can support herself by turning it into a bed-and-breakfast.

It must be acknowledged that at certain socioeconomic levels, just about all a woman can worry about is survival—decent housing, food, and keeping a job in an ageist society. Some of my subjects, however, have struggled as single mothers or lived through periods of dependency in their younger years but managed to go back to school and move on to financial independence. The plight of older women who are impoverished or sick and alone is grave and growing but too large a subject for the scope of the present book.

Whatever the status of our personal relationships, if we want to seize the day in our middle or later years—to say, *yes,* this is the time to reach for a more passionate life—we have to make important choices all over again. Here are some questions for readers so you can begin doing a self-assessment of your readiness for entering the Second Adulthood or proceeding to a more advanced phase:

a. Who am I going to be now that I'm fully grown up?
b. When will I be middle-aged?
c. When will I be old?
d. What do I like doing the best?
e. What am I doing to pursue that passion?
f. Does my present life partner offer support or resistance to that pursuit?
g. Am I still a sexual being?
h. If not, is it possible to become one again?
i. How long do I plan to live?
j. How long do I need to work?
k. Do I want to be married? Remarried?
l. If not, do I want a partner or a lover?
m. What am I doing to satisfy the longing for spiritual nourishment?
n. What will give my life meaning five years from now?
o. What will I leave behind?

Chapter 4

Pursuit of the Passionate Life

*P*assion is the central motivation of all human activity. The pursuit of a passionate life is elective, a conscious process, as opposed to the unconscious imperatives that move us, stage by stage, from childhood through adult development. And sexual revitalization is only one of three paths to a more passionate life.

As noted in the previous chapter, an equally important part of pursuing the passionate life is to find something you love to do. This is more than a search for a new hobby or a new romance. It is truly a new concept of yourself in the world, one that will generate exhilaration and commitment to the future. Even those who enjoy an exciting professional life and appear to have an enviable marriage may start feeling an indefinable itch in their fifties. Something's missing. And it's something big. It's a new dream.

The new dream will draw upon a dimension of yourself that either has fallen dormant or never was allowed full expression. You may have to reach way back into adolescence to touch it. Think of it as an activity you loved so much that hours would slip by unnoticed while it occupied you. Imagine the person that you used to dream of becoming. These reveries may appear totally impractical, especially from an income-producing standpoint. But from them may come a spark that will bring color and life's blood into your everyday existence, preventing it from becoming a long trudge down the same old road.

I bumped into an embodiment of this principle, literally, when I heard a neighbor walking ahead of me one evening on our street in New York, singing "On the Street Where You Live." She wasn't just humming, she was swinging her arms and *warbling.* Madeline is an attractive, cosmopolitan woman, a journalist and photographer, who looks to be in her late fifties and usually projects a laid-back, even jaded attitude. Why not? one would think, since she appeared to have quite a glamorous existence, living much of the time abroad with a successful husband.

What I didn't know, until I asked to interview her, was that Madeline had been depressed and in limbo for at least the past five years. It had taken her that long to extract herself from a marriage where both sex and emotional intimacy had drastically deteriorated. She had enjoyed an affair with a younger lover and survived breast cancer. She had tried living by herself in a Long Island suburb, close to her mother, after her son left for college. Valiant attempts to find a spark within the singles scene in Suffolk County had only deepened her loneliness, until it bordered on despair. At that point she had moved back to Manhattan and realized that the path out of darkness, for her, would not be through sex or romance.

"I've started taking voice lessons," she whispered when I caught up with her singing on the street. She was on her way home from a voice lesson and sounded as excited as a child. "I keep singing this song over and over and over! It's like not being able to eat enough chocolate. I began to wonder what's going on, but I guess singing was a recessed dream. I always got great pleasure from it, whether it was singing my son to sleep or singing in the car."

But when she sang, her husband and son would admonish her to be quiet so they could listen to the radio and "real professional singers." Madeline was always afraid to try out for a chorus, and it was only now, in her fifty-eighth year, that she was giving in to her core passion for expressing joy through music. She will never achieve her girlhood dream of singing backup for Stevie Wonder, of course, but that's not the point. Now when she can't sleep, she gets up in the middle of the night and practices her scales. Singing gives her physical pleasure. It has reawakened her hunger for intimacy, physical touch, someone to dance with, and she is dating again.

But what it means to anyone to find a new dream in midlife is much more elemental, and Madeline described it with unguarded delight: "It gives me a passionate thrill. I can only liken it to that feeling of when you've just met somebody. I feel like I've got a crush on singing."

◆   ◆   ◆

There is a vital link between finding the passion that will enliven the second half of your life and reopening the pathway to sexual pleasure, intimacy, and companionship. The object of both searches is the wish to reach mature love and a sense of meaning and purpose that can outlast even the death of your mate or your own demise. One often leads to, and likely accelerates, the other.

Carl Jung describes the dream in metaphysical terms: "The dream is the small hidden door in the deepest and most intimate sanctum of the soul, which opens into that primeval cosmic night that was soul long before there was a conscious ego and will be soul far beyond what a conscious ego could ever reach." It implies transcending the boundaries of self and tapping into the collective inspiration of human endeavor.

◆   ◆   ◆

If sexuality and a new dream are the first two paths, a third path to the passionate life is through spiritual exploration. In America, and most western European societies, people are led to believe that the spirit is separate from the mind and body. As a result, the spirit is an area of growth many of us set aside or compartmentalize on a single day of worship. Others find ourselves half hoping the day will come when some soul-stretching peak experience will lift us out of our ordinary consciousness for a glimpse of the sacred and eternal.

It is natural to yearn for a freeing of the spirit in our Second Adulthood. This is an ideal time to begin a program of spiritual rejuvenation, if it hasn't happened already, and to build it into our routine. We can meditate, pray, practice yoga, or even take a brisk walk twice a day and clear the mind and release those nice endorphins. Any of these is a better alternative to a cigarette, another drink, or a blowup with our partner or co-workers. And just because we might be more spiritually centered doesn't mean we have to be less sexy. In fact, the more sexually relaxed we are, the more receptive we are to all of life's pleasures—including spiritual ones.

Some people may challenge the religious proscriptions that confined them in their younger years, seeking out a more individually defined spiritual path. Others return to a more orthodox path and speak of taking a "faith walk" and becoming born again. How much thought have you given to the great metaphysical questions of life and death, faith and doubt? What do you look forward to, if anything, in the afterlife? This path requires reading, thinking, contemplation, or prayer, but it doesn't demand clear answers. The pilgrimage is the point.

We will meet divorced women whose spiritual hunger gave them the courage to turn away from censure by conservative church fathers for exploring their sexuality. We will also hear from a woman who found that the secret to saving a marriage headed for the rocks was to answer a call from God.

❖   ❖   ❖

Once you commit to pursuing the passionate life, any one of these three paths may start you off on the journey. A sexual resurgence may come first and be the stimulus for a burst of new hopes and a personal renaissance that is also spiritual. Or the decision to follow a new dream, and the wit and work it takes to build it, can generate the gradual transformation from a two-dimensional young woman into a flourishing seasoned woman. And the seasoned spiritual woman, animated as she is by a purpose beyond the maintenance of self, is a naturally seductive creature. Sex, passion, and soul go together. It's a chicken-or-egg argument.

Here is a pertinent comment from a woman in her late fifties. She found her new dream and is living in a committed relationship with a new life mate she met six years ago through a dating service. She says, "The more a woman enjoys whatever activity she is doing, the more she will radiate her joy and energy for life. This acts as a beacon that attracts people, including possible life companions."

> Do what you love
> and love will find you.

•   •   •

From studying the lives of the interviewees for this book, I discerned a pattern to the pursuit of a passionate life. There is a natural sequence to this personal renaissance, although the phases are not precisely tied to age. That is the beauty of this quest: people can begin to reach for the passionate life at any point leading up to or within their Second Adulthood.

The boldest and most fortunate people will begin preparing for their new journey in their forties, but most women won't take the time to think about reawakening to the possibilities for their own new life until they have launched their last child. Many others will need the upheaval of menopause to give them a push. Some may muddle on with the status quo into their sixties or seventies, until they are jolted by a serious illness or the wake-up call of a close contemporary's death. Or until they experience the shattering loss of a lifelong mate through divorce or death, and find themselves, perhaps for the first time, alone.

If the pursuit of a passionate life were set to music as a symphony, it would have five movements. Ideally, one would flow into the next organically. That sequence of phases is represented in the diagram at the end of this chapter. The Arc of Pursuit of the Passionate Life curves over and above the age-linked ladder of stages and Predictable Passages of Second Adulthood.

People set their own tempo for moving through these phases. Most of us are familiar by now with our own step style, the characteristic manner in which we attack the tasks of development and react to the efforts we make. Some of us take a few cautious steps ahead to test new ground, then drop back and reconsider before we get up the nerve to move forward. Others respond better to setting up sink-or-swim situations. Still others procrastinate, sticking with the status quo until life itself deals the next hand and forces a move.

Phases of the Pursuit of the Passionate Life

Phase I: *The Romantic Renaissance*

If your heart and mind are open to the idea of a personal renaissance in midlife, something or somebody will surely reawaken your senses and you will know, again, the romance of the new. The romantic rush might happen, for a married couple, on their first holiday alone together after they deposit the last child at college. The romance for a postmenopausal divorcée may begin with daring to pick up on a dream long deferred.

Whatever the source of the electricity, it is a surge that reminds a woman that she is still a woman. If she finds an outlet for this renewed energy in a new personal relationship, a new dream, or a new spiritual focus, she is on her way to pursuing a passionate life. Romantic passion offers the opportunity to live completely in the present and escape, temporarily, the baggage of the past and nagging questions of the future. While it is often short-lived, it is an exhilarating send-off to the journey of the Second Adulthood.

We will learn about the pitfalls of the Romantic Renaissance, which can be deeper and more dangerous than when we were teenagers or twenty-somethings, because we have so much more at stake. Freighting the midlife romantic fling with expectations of lasting love or marriage can end in disappointment, just as at any other life stage. Similarly, if the romance is with a new dream, it will take patience to find a practical way to integrate it into daily life.

Some women and men try to prolong this Romantic Renaissance, for years. We'll meet Sydney, a widow who fell in love with her much younger ski instructor and managed, by providing him monetary and career support, to keep him bound to her for the next twenty years, only to find herself distraught when he dropped her in her late sixties. We'll also meet Anna, a former California assemblywoman, who at 74 is still dating younger men, with no intention of going deeper. I call her Anna the Vamp of Tarzana.

Phase II: *Learning to Be Alone with Your New Self*

Once the initial passion of the romantic rush wanes, and before you can embrace your full power as a seasoned woman, you will need to spend time alone. Women need to learn how to be alone without feeling abandoned—*before* they launch their last child or perhaps find themselves without a partner. A twice-divorced journalist I met in Phoenix, now 51 and with three children still at home, is only at the beginning of this phase. "I'm reexamining everything. Who am I? Who *was* I? I don't know how much of me is even present in my life at this point." She is only now beginning to progress to thinking about the next question: "Who do I want to be?"

To answer that question, you will need to shed outgrown roles and old "shoulds" that are now superfluous, and reveal what you love about yourself and what more you might be in your own eyes and in the eyes of God.

This phase is a time to enjoy having an "affair" with yourself. Do you know how to go out to dinner alone and really enjoy it? Have you taken a trip alone and found out how to make new acquaintances? How much do you know about pleasuring yourself, sexually? Women who find themselves single in midlife, or later, will move beyond projecting desperation only after they learn to enjoy their own company.

You will have successfully moved through this phase once you are beyond expecting that a man should take care of you. The seasoned woman is attractive because she can take care of herself. Some we will hear from find they prefer to maintain a certain distance between themselves and a new lover or husband. One woman even negotiated a "postnuptial agreement" with her husband: they will live apart but commit to caring for and about each other to the end.

Learning to be with yourself also allows for growth of the mind and a widening of your imagination about the realm of future possibilities.

Phase III: *The Boldness to Dream*

As Carl Sandburg wrote, "Nothing happens unless first a dream."
Another of my favorite quotes on the subject is from Goethe,
the eighteenth-century German poet whose creativity survived
into his eighties. He expresses the spirit of this phase:

> Whatever you can do or dream you can, begin it.
> Boldness has genius, power, and magic in it.

It is interesting that the most common phrase of defiance I
hear in interviews with women who have divorced by midlife is
"I don't want to defer anymore." There is a double meaning:
They don't want to defer to a husband's wishes just because he's
the man. And they don't want to defer exploring their own
dream until it dries up for good.

We will hear from people who have found that dream within
an existing marriage. The great potential of pursuing a passionate life within a marriage or committed relationship is the joy
of sharing the work on a new dream with your partner. Single
women and men in midlife also become emboldened to think
outside the box and may begin a second act. Some formerly married, heterosexual women we will meet are exploring love and a
shared dream with another woman.

Phase IV: *Soul Seeking*

As we move into the late fifties and beyond, there is likely to be
a dramatic change in our needs and perspective. The shadow of
mortality is now prominent among the background colors of
life. As pilgrims on an uncharted path, many look toward the
light of faith. A restless soul will try out alternative spiritual
paths. Others may become more prayerful or satisfy their souls'
longing by giving back, in some way, to the next generation.

A different kind of love relationship is desired at this stage, a
deeper soul connection. The greatest boon on this journey be-

yond the conventions of First Adulthood is to connect with someone who loves and respects the pilgrim soul in you. It could be your mate, if you both appreciate each other's soul over and above your changing faces and bodies. Some of the most satisfied women in my surveys are those with lengthy marriages who have cultivated a deep soul connection with their mates; they know each other to their depths, and they know the other would be there, if necessary, to shepherd them through depression, sickness, or inconsolable loss. Most single women and men will look for someone who can be a true friend and potential partner in life, though not necessarily another marriage.

The people we will meet in this section of the book have forged soul connections in all kinds of ways—within a reinvigorated marriage, with a lover outside marriage, within a romantic friendship, or with a same-sex partner. It could be a rekindling of an old flame. But not all the rediscoveries women make in the Second Adulthood fit into a neat category. Most defy Hollywood story lines, and some defy even the words we attempt to use to describe them. I have met women who said they were having "passionate sex," though they were in fact talking about how passionate a relationship had become after the sexual side of it had been compromised by illness or tragedy.

Phase V: *Graduating to Grandlove*

This is the pot of gold at the end of the arc. If the dream of your Second Adulthood has been integrated by now with the design of your new life, you should enjoy greater confidence and self-control. If you have revived the sparks in a long marriage and accepted your differences, the ride from here on should be much smoother. Sex can also be enlivened by the simple fact of having more free time. But you don't have to be in each other's pockets. Grandlove is such a trusted affection, you don't necessarily have to live or travel together all the time.

For divorced women, even those sworn to singlehood, this older, gentler phase may change their minds and open their hearts. We will read about a widow who had a high-stepping political career but never took her eye off one of her old college boyfriends. The moment he was widowed, she pounced, and together, in their mid-sixties, they set off on a whole second round of pursuing a more passionate life together.

Grandparenthood is likely by now, bringing back a playful side. The capacity for wonder that we felt as children can be reborn through the eyes and enthusiasms of our grandchildren. Grandlove, like grandparenting, can be less about daily drudgery and more about the delights of enjoying relationships.

A broader view of life and a shorter time to live favor the growth of the Communal Heart, a form of love for the wider community expressed through giving creatively, philosophically, philanthropically, or through activism. In the Grandlove phase, one's goals are realigned with a view toward what one will leave behind. That realignment may be around a new work, idea, or purpose, a renewed faith, or a deeper love.

But Grandlove doesn't have to be confined to doing good in the manner of a chaste church lady. There is another role for older women: that of a Seasoned Siren. These women are able to enchant both older and younger men into feeling like boys again because they know the secrets of seduction. It's the ultimate head trip, dependent not on beauty or youth but on vitality, wit, sass, and the cultivated ability to tell a good story, energize men's egos, and alternate between maternal warmth and sexual sizzle.

Pursuit of the Passionate Life

Phase III
Boldness to Dream

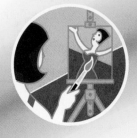

Phase II
Learning to Be Alone

Phase I
Romantic Renaissance

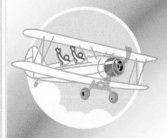

Passage to the Age of Mastery

Selective
60s

Feisty
50s

Pits to Peak

Age 45 ⟶ 49

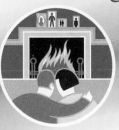

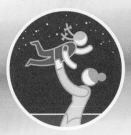

Passage to Cultivation or Isolation

Ascent to
Centenarian

Passage to the Age of Unity

Enduring
80s

Noble
90s

Spontaneous
70s

Predictable
Passages of
Second Adulthood

Chapter 5

The Sexual Path

*N*ow we are ready to take a look at people who are trying out each of the three different paths that can start us off on pursuing a more passionate life. In the next four chapters, you are invited to sit in on my group interviews with real-life, down-to-earth women and men.

A Big Woman

Carole Smith is not young, not thin, not rich, and not gorgeous, but she is one of the most sensual and satisfied midlife women I met in the course of my research. "Dating over fifty is great," she enthused in one of the first group interviews I held with women 50 and over, this one at a Health and Healing Center in Red Bank, New Jersey. "I'm looking for fun and companionship and romance—"

Before she could finish, another woman interrupted: "You don't go as far as sex?"

"Oh, I have a lot of sex," Carole said, her voluptuous chest rippling with her hearty laughter.

It isn't the first guess one would make about Carole. She is a 50-year-old manager of a doctor's office who has been divorced for more than twenty years. She describes herself as "a big, bubbly, fun-loving Jersey girl." Her face is an inviting smile, even in repose, her hair subtly tinted auburn and cut in a simple, flattering way to frame her broad face. She loves putting on makeup because it transforms her from plain to pretty. Her naturally full body is probably fifty pounds over the national standard for her medium height. Yet Carole is a walking advertisement for the joys of what I call "middlesex." When she is asked how sex has changed for her from 40 to 50, she tosses her hair and grins. "Better. Why? I don't have to worry about getting pregnant. I didn't have the same trouble separating the 'mother me' from the 'sexual me' once I launched my child. If you're a sensual person, by the time you're fifty, you've become much better at it. You can bring a man to his knees, and it's not even hard. I love dating in my fifties. It can be just about you and him."

Carole had a lot of lost time to make up for, having married at the age of 19 in the hunger to have a child to love her. Her husband was a good man, a police officer, but emotionally remote. At 22, this good Catholic mom was separated and left alone with a 2-year-old boy. The struggle of mothering while working full-time to make ends meet and juggling the parenting with her son's father drained her energies. Her desire for men and sex fell dormant, not just temporarily but for the next twenty years. She watched the wretchedness of women whose self-worth was wholly dependent on whether or not they had a man in their lives; no, not for her. Carole put her emphasis instead on finding satisfaction in a job where she made herself indispensable, spending quiet hours in solitude getting to know herself, and seeking sensual pleasure in eating and drinking with friends.

And then one day, there she was, sitting with her mother at Mass, of all places, when it changed. The priest was too virile, too carelessly seductive behind his safe white collar, to inspire only chaste thoughts. "He's really cute," she whispered to her mother, who rolled her eyes. "Carole Ann!"

"Oh, my!" Carole chuckled to herself, feeling a tingle run through her 42-year-old body. "I guess I'm attracted to men again."

She decided to start dating, but how? She went out and bought a new computer and asked for instruction from her son on how to access the Internet. There were no online dating services at the time, but she logged on to a New Jersey chat room for divorced people. "The first man I met online was pivotal in my life," she says, but when he asked her for a picture she backed off. He pressed to meet her in person. She confessed she was afraid to meet and that she was, well, oversized.

"Hey," he responded, "I'm a big guy. My ex-wife was big. I like big." He was a police officer like her first husband, six foot six, and Carole says she will love that man forever. Unfortunately, she admits, she zeroed in on him as her next husband. Weighting the relationship with all her repressed desires of two decades, it collapsed. "Even though it didn't work out, he got me out of the house," she says with the hindsight that followed the heartbreak. "That was his role. So I honor him. The universe sent me exactly what I needed—not a husband, not a soulmate, but *knowledge.*"

On Top of the Ladder of Life

Women who are *un*married in middle or later life, like Carole, are no longer on the sad fringes of society. According to a 2003 AARP study of lifestyles and dating among midlife singles, most older single women feel they are "on top of the ladder of life." Whether they're in their fifties, sixties, or seventies, they are generally upbeat. Both midlife men and women love the freedom that being single brings—citing independence, getting to keep their houses however they want, and not having to compromise with another person. The downside, especially for women, is that they often find themselves wanting someone to talk to and do things with.

But midlife divorce does not need to signal the beginning of an eternity alone. The proof is in another stunning finding from the AARP divorce study:

> 75% of women who divorced in their 50s reported enjoying a serious, exclusive relationship after their divorces, sometimes as early as within two years. Among men, 81% reported the same agreeable outcome.

Fortunately, today a single woman over 50 doesn't need to belly up at a singles' bar to meet someone. She can find an age-specific date just by moving a computer mouse in her own house.

"The old excuse—'I just can't meet anyone'—doesn't fly in the age of online dating," asserts Carole Smith. "It's like going to the candy store. If you don't like what you've picked, you just reach back into the jar. The Internet is a candy jar full of a million men!"

While the buzz and expectations surrounding online dating have died down among the broad population, the playing field it has opened up for older women remains a bonanza. It has changed the arena of possibilities more than any other factor. Those who have tried online dating say they can find out more about a man by exchanging ten e-mails with him than by going out on a couple of dates. Online socializing has made it easier for those who want to slow down the dating/mating protocol to more like it was before the sexual revolution. And that gives women more power and protection. The Web allows for anonymity and invisibility and allows women to initiate contact. If at any point an online correspondent turns them off, they have a quick escape: simply clicking the "Block User" button makes him disappear forever.

Janet Lever, a sociologist at California State University, Los Angeles, has done a study of online dating with fifteen thousand respondents for *ELLE*/MSNBC.com. She found that nearly 50 percent of the women users say they are getting more dates, more sex, and more lasting love as a result of using online personals. Only 36 percent of men note a positive change in their social life when dating online. Lever's study also revealed that women in their forties and fifties, who often have a tough time finding the right someone in the real world, are the age group having the most luck in the virtual world.

"After nearly forty years of women's liberation, women still don't typically ask men out," says Lever. "But in the virtual world, they do. It shows a huge shift in women's ability to initiate socially and sexually."

Dating Can Change Your Self-Image

While women beyond 45 have been told for a long time that their bodies become invisible to men, at least some of them are regaining confidence in their natural contours at this age. Carole Smith, for one, is no longer self-conscious about her full figure. She has learned how to put her assets to use. "If a man knows he's going to be pleasured—and you make sure he gets pleasure right away—he's not going to be grading you on your body shape," she says, adding frankly, "Men are really just interested in your breasts and your butt."

Like most of the divorced women in their fifties whom I have interviewed, it took Carole a while to get beyond the husband-hunting agenda. The two men she really wanted both rejected her after the idyllic stage of their romances. She had to work hard to change her attitude about rejection.

"Sometimes a romance and a breakup can be the best thing that can happen," she says now. Carole has had one relationship of two years, another that almost turned into an engagement, and her current lover, with whom she has been enjoying passionate romantic love for the last two years. "Men are fun! I celebrate the differences." What she finds most important is retaining the friendship when the romantic flame goes out. As she wisely observes, "Relationships change. Just because a dating relationship didn't work out romantically, so what? There's much more to life, and friendship is always first and last with me."

Several years ago she faced probably the worst trauma a woman can imagine: her son, her only child, died of a fatal heart arrhythmia. Her ex-husband gave a beautiful eulogy. But what truly buoyed her came from a surprise source, a delta of loving friendships: three of her former lovers came to the wake and funeral.

Carole has developed a truly seasoned woman's philosophy of life: "I may never get that perfect soulmate. But you know what?" She raises her glass of sparkling water and rolls her eyes. "I'm gonna have a hell of a time trying."

Having survived tragedy, Carole is able to distinguish between heartbreak and mere heartache. "I never do romantic drama," she says. "I don't get into 'Oh, he doesn't like me, I'm devastated.' " Here is the distinction she makes, a distinction worth remembering: "9/11 was devastating. Losing your child is devastating. Losing a man is *not* devastating. You save devastated for cancer."

The Midlife Singles Explosion

Why so much traffic in the midlife singles bazaar? Part of it is the sociology of the boomer generation. In 1996, a very significant spike in divorce was recorded by the U.S. Census Bureau among women and men who were born between 1945 and 1954. Divorce peaked among these earliest boomers—men and women who are today (in 2006) between the ages of 51 and 60—exactly the age group moving into their seasoned years. Forty-one percent of men who are today in their fifties have been divorced at some point, as have 39 percent of women in the same age group. Many of these are the people who were socialized during the sexual revolution to believe that divorce is healthier than a miserable marriage—especially an unequal one. (Happily, the proportion of marriages breaking up has been declining in the United States since 1980 as people marry later and delay the responsibilities of parenthood.)

Another startling change is in who is asking for the divorce. Demographers note a spike in divorces among women who are now in their early to mid-forties. This is when most of us first sense the advancing shadow of midlife and register the "hurry-up feeling" that is almost universal at this stage. Among women in the AARP divorce study who left their first marriages anytime between the ages of 40 and 74, almost three quarters split during their forties. Many remain single and move into and out of serial relationships. A snapshot of this startlingly new and fluid playing field was revealed in the 2004 study of divorce at midlife by the AARP.

Two thirds of divorces among couples over age 40 are *initiated* by the wives.

One third of divorced or single women over 40 are dating younger men—a reversal of past behavior.

The single woman in her fifties is much more likely today to be divorced or never married than widowed.

These feisty boomer women show every indication of looking forward to courtship, romance, and love as a normal part of middle and later life. In the past this might have been true only for the glamorous, powerful, or bohemian sets.

Why are wives the ones most likely today to precipitate a midlife divorce?

Because they can.

What has changed just as dramatically as longevity is that women today in their fifties, sixties, even seventies are likely to be holding down good jobs. Since women's career aspirations are often delayed or interrupted by child rearing, their professional lives may be only starting or, very likely, still expanding in their Second Adulthood. Their excitement expands apace. Their husbands, usually older and having had a head start, are more likely to be slowing down, topped off in their careers, or laid off in the push by corporate America to trim high-salaried veterans from its workforce. Many men in their late fifties or early sixties, fit and fidgety, are moping around at home in sweatpants.

Why do women stay in unsatisfying marriages for so long? The number one reason they give is "because of the children." Another reason, given by one quarter of the over-40 women in the AARP study, was that they needed time to prepare financially; otherwise they couldn't afford to get divorced. That helps to explain a line I often heard from my interviewees: "I left the marriage, in spirit, five years before I walked out the door."

I know what some readers are probably thinking at this point: *I'm never going to be a poster girl for dating and sex after 50, because I'm never going to leave him.* The lives of women like Bebe or Carole may seem quite daring compared to your life. But there are many other women we will meet in this book who are finding their own less dramatic ways to mature into seasoned women. Some are able to do it within an existing relationship, others by taking the plunge into divorce.

When Push Comes to Shove

What prods women to divorce in middle or later life is not likely to be some self-indulgent whim; it is usually a chronic problem that has become intolerable. Pam's story is typical of women who lose themselves in the First Adulthood under the weight of a traditional, patriarchal marriage. Pam was part of a group of older, married, suburban women in Stamford, Connecticut, who spontaneously gathered with me after an author's luncheon at a large public library, eager to talk about their experiences with love, sex, divorce, and dating.

Pam is a born extrovert, with a broad mouth, a bass voice, and a generous disposition. She had resisted marriage in her young years and gotten by in a series of office jobs. In fact, she confessed, she really got married, at age 42, out of fear of being alone in middle age—and it was out of fear that she remained married until it hurt.

"Being an old-style Italian man, my husband's attitude was 'I go to work, I come home, that's it,' but I guess I wanted someone to take care of," Pam admits with hindsight, "so I was the one who came home from work and did the washing and cleaning." The other women in her group groan; so typical. Pam shrugs. "Before I married him, I was a fun-loving, extroverted, bubbly person. But with him, I lost my identity. My oldest friend kept saying, 'Where did Pam go?' "

Then her mate blatantly admitted that he was seeing another woman. It was the girl he worked with, a decade younger than Pam. He said he didn't want the affair to break up their marriage and that he would end it.

"Of course," chime in the other women, "they always say that."

Pam admits that she put up with it for four more years, determined to fix the marriage as she had fixed everything else. She gave him her last best effort at ardent sex. Then her friend saw an episode of *Judge Judy* and told Pam, "You're an enabler."

"What's that?"

"You're enabling him to keep this double life going." Pam realized that her husband, too weak to leave himself, wanted her to kick him out. When he rented a house for his playmate, Pam finally had enough. The marriage ended with a whimper.

In divorces initiated by the wives, the evidence is strong that without painful action taken by the woman, a husband's grievous behavior would not have stopped. The number one reason given by women in the AARP study for why they sought divorce was verbal, physical, or emotional abuse (23%). After that came alcoholism or drug abuse (18%) and marital cheating (17%). Not what one would call minor annoyances.

Six months after her separation, Pam tells us, she went to her gynecologist for a checkup.

"What's up?" the doctor asked as she inserted the speculum. "You're not even flinching."

"It's been a long time—even *this* is beginning to feel good!" That story brought amused hoots from our group.

While awaiting her divorce, Pam lost her job and had to scale down to a one-bedroom apartment. One night, a former co-worker, a very much younger man, dropped by. After they'd had a few drinks, he offered himself as a "friend with benefits." They went to bed and—voilà! It was a whole lot more fun than the speculum. "It was good sex, and it made me want more," Pam recalls. More of life, as well as sex.

Her divorce had become final only a year before she told us this story. Gingerly, she admits to being 53 now. "*Are* we that old? We don't feel it. My friend with benefits taught me a lot. Especially oral sex—I used to be turned off by that. He laughed at me because I'd say, 'Oooh, this is fun! I never knew about this!' "

For Pam, the most important benefit of her divorce and sexual revitalization is the recovery of her identity. "Pam's back!" She shimmies a little. "A lonely Pam, but that's more easily rectified than being in a bad marriage and losing yourself. My new policy is 'Go everywhere you're invited!' I am going out with friends more and more, both work and personal, I'm trying Internet dating, and I'm hoping to meet someone who will mean something!"

It is the confidence and newfound freedom Pam discovered, once she got beyond the fear of being alone, that soon led her to a new vocation: administrator at a large and popular library. Pam grins. "They said they wanted someone crazy and extroverted—that's the real me." In her new position, she deals not only with her three bosses but with the entire library staff as well. This allows her to work as the congenital nurturer but also to let her exuberant personality loose.

"I love it!" Pam exclaims. "I'll be there till the day I die. Libraries are very nurturing. And having a job you like is huge. Especially when you're single and older and you don't have any family support."

The progression that Pam describes is revealing. After finally reaching the limit of her tolerance for chronic unfaithfulness and taking the rough consequences of divorce, she spent time learning to be alone, then allowed herself a spree of sexual spontaneity. Her sexual revival gave her the boost of self-confidence to recapture her identity and led to a new vocation. Working for a library may seem too tame to call "a dream," but to Pam, it's a dream job.

Chapter 6

The Dream Path

A second potent path to a more passionate life begins with discovering your new dream. The activity that will ignite new passion in your Second Adulthood does not always manifest itself easily. Hampered by obligations and responsibilities, many of us have forgotten, by midlife, what it was that we used to love to do most. To find that source of joy requires a concrete commitment to change things in a way that will rebuild our enthusiasm for life. The discovery process needs to be something we think about every day, talk about, meditate on, dream about, argue over and laugh about with a mate or friends. Then one day the *Aha!* moment hits, and the reaction will probably be "Oh, of course."

After the first glimpse of the new dream comes the commitment to pursue it with one's full heart and mind. And that may require a major restructuring of one's life to build a new foundation.

My own eyes were opened to the life-changing potential of a new dream when I gathered with a group of unconventional women in San Francisco. We met in a cozy beauty salon presided over by Marlene Mendieta, a former high-salaried bond trader. When the financial market bubble burst, she saw her job evaporate, her company go down, and her colleagues scatter. An assisted blonde with a vague resemblance to Marilyn Monroe, Marlene maintains an upbeat view of life and radiates youthful energy, accented by her bouncy ponytail. Not many of her acquaintances know that she has been widowed for many years.

When she lost her job, Marlene was stunned, alone, and at a loss for what to do next. Making money for rich clients had lost its appeal. But she loved doing hair. And she needed to meet new people. Marlene was willing to live much more frugally in order to play out her secret fantasy. Ignoring her snobbier friends' disparaging remarks, she leased a cozy space in an alley just off a fashionable San Francisco street of boutiques and invited everyone she knew to come for a haircut and to bring their dogs.

In the last few years, Marlene's dream has become reality. Her place has evolved into a special kind of community, less a shop than a social salon. "I'm not the best hairdresser, but it's the package," as Marlene says. The atmosphere is both homey, with pet beds everywhere, and retroromantic, with oversized photos of James Dean and Marilyn Monroe adorning the walls. Women drop by at the end of the day to have a glass of wine, share their stories, and enjoy some TLC.

When eight of us met there after hours, the regulars drew up a sofa and barber chairs and sat with their twitchy Lhasas and cuddly cockers ladled into their laps. The first to tell her story was Marlene's sister, Carlene.

"Making love with Walt is like doing barrel rolls in an open-cockpit Piper Cub," says Carlene, laughing as she shakes out her freshly shampooed red hair. "We fly together too," she explains, "in a little aerobatic biplane."

"You don't do aerobatics in an open cockpit, do you?" asks one of the older married women.

"Sure, we take turns at the controls," Carlene says. "One of us is flying and the other is laughing and holding on to Rosey, the dog."

Bernice applauds. "Just keep flying!" she counsels. "It's like dancing. It keeps you young."

Bernice's voice is able to run sultry or cool. By day, she assumes the bristly manner of a career bureaucrat, but her nighttime persona is flauntingly seductive, with moves mastered as a competitive ballroom dancer. She proudly describes how she keeps her lover at bay. "I'm not ready for marriage yet," she insists. "My current man even asked his mother to intercede. She had me over for tea and asked me to marry him. But I'm much too independent, it would ruin the relationship."

Sam, an extrovert with a husky voice and a sharp tongue who enjoys shocking her uptight WASP family, strokes her Tibetan spaniel and offers her own recipe for avoiding prolonged entanglement with men: "A woman's best friend is a dog. Dogs don't judge you, they never leave you, and *they* don't leave wet spots on the bed."

It might sound like Carrie, Samantha, Charlotte, and Miranda dishing on *Sex and the City.* Except that all the women in this group were over 50—some way over. Marlene is 55. Carlene is 50. Sam is 67. Bernice is 88. Aging has not dimmed their dreams. On the contrary, it has emboldened them to take leaps of imagination beyond the usual earthly conventions.

The Sky's the Limit

Carlene, for instance, who loves doing aerobatics with her lover either in bed or several thousand feet up in the air, is a dental surgeon with three marriages behind her who recently celebrated her fiftieth birthday. As a girl, she had thrilled to the legend of Amelia Earhart, but in the Nevada mining town where she grew up poor, the dream of flying was as remote as the possibility of going to college—though she eventually managed to do both. To stave off a midlife crisis, she started taking flying lessons in her mid-forties. By then, her dental practice was settled down to three and a half days a week and she thought, "I have the money and time now—here we go!"

Her flight instructor was impressed that she wanted to learn on a Piper Cub, the airplane equivalent of a Model T Ford. She and Walt soon discovered they shared a sense of adventure and a love of antique planes. Carlene's microscopic world, staring into oral cavities all day, was expanded once Walt introduced her to the vastness of the skies over Sonoma's vineyards. At a hundred feet in the air they could see San Francisco, at a thousand feet the Pacific, and on a clear day all the way to the High Sierras.

"It's totally freeing," says Carlene.

The pursuit of her dream of flying led her to a place beyond her wildest imagination—into a love affair with her 22-year-old flight instructor. Walt is a quarter century her junior. Their mutual attraction grew out of their shared passion. Carlene was the only "girl" who hung around the Sonoma Sky Park, where, she laughs, "It's always hot and dusty and windy and you look like shit." But to Walt, a youthful man with a broad grin, Carlene, in her tank tops, jeans, and motorcycle boots, was incredibly sexy, the focus of all the older men—"the trophy girl." Up in the air, her professional status fell away and she was dependent on him to learn how to land into the wind. On the ground, he was the more off-balance one, seeing a therapist to guide him through the uncertainties of his twenties.

The chemistry they felt went beyond a defiance of age and social norms. "She'd call and want to go flying at six A.M. and she'd want to fly until six P.M.," Walt told me in a follow-up interview, "and you don't get that kind of energy out of most people." They were both beguiled by the romance of early aviation: no rules, no restraints, just flying free as a bird. Walt coached her so well that once she was licensed, Carlene was chosen to fly a replica of Amelia Earhart's legendary 1927 open-cockpit plane in an air show. Lean and leggy, her coppery-red hair tucked up under a vintage helmet, she zigzagged, alone, from New York to Los Angeles and back, putting down after seventy-three hours of piloting a plane as flimsy as a packing box.

"It takes a great pilot to do that," Walt told me, his neck puffing up with pride. Carlene was her instructor's romantic fantasy. And he was hers.

Sharing her dream with an adoring young man made everything about it rapturously romantic. Carlene smiles at Walt's description of the sensation of doing cockpit barrel rolls. "You can go hang upside down by your seat belts, or you can do smooth, old-time acrobatics," Walt says. "It's like ballroom dancing in the Thirties and Forties." That's the kind of reference that prompts her to describe her young partner as "an old soul."

Carlene is more of a risk taker than most, but she embodies several important elements that characterize the seasoned woman, who is most likely to be working, proud of achieving economic independence, and fiercely protective of her hard-earned status.

Step by step, through the course of her three marriages, Carlene worked hard to build an independent identity, going back to school to pursue a profession that would allow her to become self-supporting.

Starting at the bottom as a dental assistant, she earned the credentials to become a doctor of periodontics. Now, at the age of 50, a serious and successful professional, she is able to indulge herself in the romantic fantasy of adolescent love with a young man who reignites her fire. And she is fearless. What's left to fear when you have survived the passages of your First Adulthood and made it over the hump of midlife? Of course, we all harbor fears of aging, destitution, death. But people who are not inhibited by those natural human anxieties are those able to live every day to the fullest—risks and all.

The dentist and the flyboy first developed a friendship, and that is key. Their friendship evolved so naturally that is was fun just to go grocery shopping together. Their social circle consists of other flying enthusiasts and the artisans who help them find and rebuild vintage planes. By now Carlene has been with Walt for five years, and she makes no apologies for it. "People told me if I dated someone that young, I'd come unglued," she recalls. "But we have a deep connection. My life feels like it's in reverse. I married men I don't think I was well matched with, and now I find the one I am well matched with and I won't marry."

The not-so-odd couple recently bought a little house together and shared the cost of an exquisite, silvery, all-aluminum vintage biplane. They spend weekends in her private hangar tinkering with Carlene's three other planes and bed down in an air-conditioned loft inside the hangar built by Walt's friends from the contracting firm for which he works. Carlene has a simple explanation for why this unconventional partnership works: "We really like each other. The fact that we happen to like a lot of the same things is a bonus. It's really the key to life. Because when you get through lusting, you've got to have something to talk about!"

When I visited the hangar on a Sunday afternoon, Walt told me that he can't imagine a future without Carlene. He insisted that he, like she, doesn't want children. Whether or not that is true remains to be seen; Walt was the one who cradled Carlene's new puppy in his arms and worried about whether they had remembered to bring her kibbles. Walt's mother dropped by and hugged Carlene, her peer, like a sister, seeming entirely comfortable with this unconventional match.

But Carlene has no illusions. "It's not likely to last. If it goes away,

I'll be extremely sad," she told the group gathered in her sister's beauty salon. Then she smiled contentedly and tossed her copper hair. "But whatever it is, it's terrific."

And whenever it ends, she will still have her dream. Carlene's love of flying is a passion that will never go away. And if the barrel rolls of her late-adolescent affair slow down, maybe she will find another flying enthusiast to share her passion.

To Leap or Not to Leap?

In the back of the mind of any woman in a tenuous marriage as she approaches 50, or later, is "Shall I resign myself to what I have? Or take the leap and see what's out there?" A surprisingly large number of the hundreds of women I queried in the course of my research were WMDs—Women Married, Dammit!—whose answer to "How do you feel about love over 50?" was "Hungry" or "Oh, I remember that" or "Never give up." Many expressed a wish to be free to date or the temptation to have a love affair with a younger man. But before they make a move, they want to know what's on the other side: *Will I find interesting men? Will they be attracted to a middle-aged woman with cellulite and droopy boobs? Or will I be sitting home with a hot toddy and cold heart watching* Sex and the City *reruns?* These women are not ready or willing to consider forfeiting the apparent security of a basically empty midlife marriage—not unless they can be guaranteed a better deal outside. That is a guarantee no one can offer.

On the day our group met in Marlene's salon, one of the regulars had suggested I pick up her friend Yvette along the way. "I'm married and wondering whether I should be," she told me right off the bat. "I'm fifty-four now, and I'm trying to figure out whether this is the way I want the rest of my life to be colored." Interesting choice of words: I had wondered, on our drive to the salon, about the color of her hair. Yvette had said, "Oh, I'm just trying to keep it from being gray." It was more like colorlessly ungray. Her skin was pale and without much makeup. She mopped her cheeks; she mentioned that she's been suffering from hot flashes for the last seven years but said she hasn't gotten around to doing anything about it. Although she's an active bicyclist and thin, she did not move with vitality. Most everything about Yvette seemed drained of color, except for two things. When she spoke of her daughters who are off in college, her voice was animated. And when she showed me the cliff-side home that she has completely redesigned since her children left, turning it into a staggered series of glass doors and serene terraced gardens, there were hints of a new dream as a landscape designer.

When we gather in the salon, she tells us that she's been married since she was 22. "I've done the old-fashioned thing of staying with somebody for so long, it's hard for me to imagine being by myself. I just really like physical contact."

Marlene, the single salon owner, nudges her: "Do you get that from your husband, though?"

"No. I would like piles of contact. I remember in the movie *Tom Jones,* Squire Weston sleeps under a whole pile of beagles. I'd like that. I'd like to sleep in a whole pile of people or animals or something. I really like contact." Some of the other women hug their lapdogs to their breasts, nodding in empathy.

Sam, the sassy WASP lady of 67 who enjoys being rebellious, states the problem: "Yvette's really fighting a battle with herself."

Yvette agrees. "It's kind of like graduating from college again. A whole new phase, a new chapter. Would it be better to leave him? I don't know. He's very depressive, so he's a big energy drain, and yet he's not a bad person. We're not fighting like cats and dogs. There's nothing that forces it to happen."

"He doesn't have any reason to change," Sam points out.

"Do you feel like it's your mission in life to be his support system?" Marlene asks.

"He does value me," Yvette says defensively. "Even if he's not particularly nice towards me, I know I'm important to him."

"Like a nurse?"

That stops Yvette for a moment. Then she laughs. "Yeah, I guess so. It answers my security needs. And I get to live in this nice house that I built. And I love it when the kids come home. If we split up, I'd only get to spend half the time with them."

Sam poses a simple, penetrating question: "When you wake up in the morning, how do you feel? Half full? Empty?"

"I feel discouraged with myself for not having gotten out of the situation," Yvette confesses.

"Every morning?" prods Sam.

"Yeah. My days feel productive and good, and I get to bike. But every day that goes by, I feel bad that I haven't gotten myself out of there."

Melanie Horn, a San Francisco psychologist, asks her, "Do you ever give yourself credit for keeping the whole thing going?"

Tellingly, Yvette doesn't seem to hear that question. What she really wants is a reassurance that nobody can give her: "I want to feel that there's definitely something better out there, so that it's an intelligent move to let go of what I have," she tells us.

By this point, we are in full amateur group therapy mode, and I can't help joining in. "It sounds like you have just defined for yourself a reason that you will always have to stay in the same situation. I'm not saying you should or shouldn't jump. You can do as much research as you like, you can do a little experimentation, you might even have a trial separation, but no one can assure you that on the other side of making the jump, you will land safely and happily and be glad that you did it. Otherwise, it wouldn't be a risk."

Now Carlene, the aviatrix, offers the benefit of her own experience: "I was married for ten years. When you make the decision to get out, for one solid year you're not going to be very happy. You're not going to be sure it was the right decision. It's going to be befuddling. But when the smoke clears at the end of that year, you won't believe you thought about *not* getting out. You'll go, 'Oh my God, what a weight gone.' "

Carlene offers her projection: "If you stepped away, that might be the impetus for him to say, 'I'm going to get some counseling,' or 'I'm going to get on medication.' He might become a person that you can have a life with. But right now, he has absolutely no reason to change." Carlene was dead right. In almost any chronically troubled relationship, often nothing changes until one partner shakes up the status quo by drawing the line: "I'm not willing to put up with this situation anymore. You have two choices—either change [and set a deadline] or you'll lose me and all the perks that go with me."

By now everyone was piling on Yvette. The arguments were so overwhelming that she was wilting, and I felt a little sorry for her. Yvette had never taken up much room in her own life. She had lost her mother as a young child and was fearful of abandonment. She needed to talk to a therapist. But the most important thing she was missing, in my view, had not been mentioned: a new dream. Even if her husband snapped out of his funk, he wouldn't be able to supply that for her. Yvette had no central focus in her life beyond her frustrations. Rather feebly, she acknowledged as much.

"I need to find some kind of career that I want to really throw myself into big time. It's embarrassing to talk about this situation in front of other people," she said, "because I realize how much it sounds like it needs to change. When you're alone, you can just normalize whatever you live with."

"In a group like this, you shouldn't feel at all vulnerable," Sam reassured her. "You just haven't expanded. You haven't developed your own passions. So the hollowness of what you are living right now is magnified."

At this stage, Yvette could be called an SQ—a Status Quo. She finds it easier to rationalize living with what she has rather than insisting upon change or making the effort to find a new dream. But during the discussion a flush of color had come up in her cheeks. Maybe it was the wine; more likely it was her reaction to the affectionate embrace of a group of women, which had accomplished its usual magic. She said later it had been as helpful as group therapy. A few years down the road, Yvette might well become a Passionate.

By this time, everyone was ready to have another glass of wine and talk about their pets. But the evening wasn't over yet.

The Octogenarian Tease

Bernice calls us to attention by banging her cane on the floor. Having listened with detached amusement to our debate about whether or not to hang on to a tattered marriage, she now cuts in.

"Who needs it?" Bernice has chosen to remain single—and singularly in command of her life and career—for all of her 88 years. That choice, she says, has hardly deprived her of male companionship; she stores more boyfriends in her memory bank than she can recall. "The one man

I really did want to marry was killed on a motorcycle a few months after we were engaged," she tells us.

We all groan. Bernice shucks off our sympathy. "No man could have put up with me. In my job with the federal government I traveled eighty percent of the time." In the 1930s and '40s, Bernice was also a champion ballroom dancer. It shows in the grace and agility she still possesses. Slender in her St. John pantsuit, her silky white hair brilliant against the forest green ensemble, Bernice is still stringing along the most persistent of her boyfriends, who is considerably younger. Fifteen years ago, when his mother interceded, Bernice was 73. The man's mother confessed that she didn't have much longer to live and would be greatly comforted if Bernice would marry her son.

"No, Thula!" Bernice stamps her cane on the floor, acting out the scene for us. "I'm not ready for marriage yet."

The ladies of the salon are amused. "Even his mom, his dying mom, couldn't capture you," giggles one of the women. The poor man has never been married. We all opined, "Bernice, what a heartbreaker!"

Ah, but that may be what has kept their romance throbbing for fifty years. The most famous seductresses and courtesans have always been elusive and resistant to being tied down, which kept the mystery alive.

Bernice and her longest-lasting lover had a fully sexual relationship until she was 79. The lapse of sex since then has not discouraged her companion. "We still kiss and all that," she says modestly. "He still calls me three times a week when we're apart. We play golf and he takes me to dinner, and we just have a wonderful time together." What they have become to each other transcends sex. They are soulmates. "He's there for me and I'm there for him, to the end," she says. "You see, we understand each other very well."

The evening in the salon was a vivid reminder of how dramatically women's roles are changing, especially after the family stage. Seasoned women no longer have to be the *über*-mother/wives, defined more by the sacrifices they make than the actions they take. The great promise of a Second Adulthood is the chance to realize their full capabilities, not just for the benefit of a husband and family but for themselves and all those they touch and inspire in the wider world.

Chapter 7

Heartland Women
Rediscovering Sex and Dreams

*J*ust how widespread is the desire for reawakening in the second half of a woman's life? I began to wonder after spending the first months of research with groups of infuriatingly fit and healthy women from California and groups of sophisticated women in New York and New Jersey. Maybe this phenomenon of women over 50 seeking sex and romance was limited only to the more permissive parts of the United States. Were women in the heartland just as bold?

After more group discussions and many more lengthy personal interviews, I decided to take a road trip across the country. Women who had corresponded with me online were eager and excited about gathering groups of their friends. As I traveled across the great and varied landscape of America, interviewing seasoned women in their forties, fifties, sixties, seventies, and eighties, in the big cities and rural heartland, I heard a common refrain. The women routinely describe the *Aha!* moment sometime in their late forties or early fifties when they realize, "I don't have a new dream." Madeline, the New York divorcée who decided to pursue her love of singing at the age of 57, and Carlene Mendieta from the last chapter, who learned to fly in her mid-forties, both realized it and acted on it.

Many other conventional women are now recognizing that if they don't work at finding a new outlet to reawaken their energies, the long day's journey ahead may be one hard, lonely slog along a flat highway (except where it's increasingly torn up for maintenance work). In fact, the ideal time for women to stage personal revolutions—sexual, emotional, spiritual—is after 50, and these revolutions can be accomplished either inside or outside a marriage.

There are many other women who have been burned by marriage and are unable to shake off the status of victim. Or they are unwilling to learn from the failure or just tired of faking loveless orgasms for too many years. These are the women who tell me, "Been there, done that, I'm so glad not to be married." Women unwilling to scroll through Internet dating sites are likely to say, "They're all leftovers and losers out there" or "There's nobody out there for a woman my age." Again and again in my group interviews those old clichés were proven wrong.

Perhaps the most surprising of these groups, however, was in the Deep South, where I hadn't expected to find middle-aged divorcées and widows overturning the conventions that used to confine such women to gossiping, grandmothering, and going to church.

Texas Women Talk Back

A group of feisty Texas women who gathered over brunch one Sunday in Fort Worth, Texas, was proof positive that things are changing fast for educated women in the South. All eight of the women had started out on the most conventional of paths—too late for the first sexual revolution—but each had challenged conventional wisdom and staged a personal revolution in midlife.

Fort Worth, the older sister city to Dallas, was an ideal window into the lives of affluent women trying to make the most of their bonus decades while going against the grain of groupthink. All the women in this gathering had had to struggle with rejection or ridicule for defining their own truths against rigid social codes and paternalistic churches. I was continually reminded, "Down here, you're fighting another whole layer—the conservative religious layer."

Historically, Fort Worth is grounded in oil money and, more recently, in computer-based wealth. Although it has a beautiful and culturally rich downtown, built mostly by the fabulous wealth of the Bass family, its communities are socially segmented in the extreme. People in the rich white sections take much of their social status from belonging to country clubs. The black and Hispanic sections are far less favored, with teachers who often spend their own money just to provide paper, pencils, and books for their students.

Sandy McCall, a silver-haired psychotherapist, suggested that her friend Darlene would make an especially illuminating addition to our group. She described her divorced friend with amazement and perhaps a smidgeon of envy: "She used to be a well-to-do west side socialite until she was dumped for the proverbial younger woman. But let me tell you— Darlene's so cute and bubbly blond and she's *out there*—she has men circling around her like sharks."

What was it really like "out there"? We were about to find out.

✦   ✦   ✦

Darlene's blond-streaked hair is still wet when she joins us at brunch. She has just jumped out of the pool at her sister's country club and thrown on shorts and a hooded sweater. She looks like a grown-up Barbie doll, but beneath the packaging there is a painfully forged inner strength. In this safe circle, Darlene Cozby tells us the inside story.

Pregnancy at 17 short-circuited her education, and, to finish high school while supporting her daughter and herself, Darlene went to work and night school. Five years after high school graduation, she married a "catch" and lived for twenty years cocooned inside his affluent, high-status world on the west side of Fort Worth, chauffeuring her three children to private schools. That external structure crumbled when her husband discarded her for a girl toy when she was in her mid-forties with only a high school degree.

"I came out of my marriage with the sexual confidence of a goober," she says. "That's a southern expression for a peanut," she explains for my benefit. She recalls the shame and self-recriminations of that period. "I couldn't imagine taking off my clothes in front of any man who hadn't slept with me for the past ten years." Beyond her degraded self-image, she had to learn how to regain self-respect in a social milieu that forgets divorcées as easily as unclaimed baggage. Darlene spells out a bald truth: "Socially, here in Fort Worth, it's much more acceptable for your husband to die than for you to divorce. At least you know that at his funeral you'll be given support. But if you're divorced, you carry a sense of shame, as if you did something wrong. You just have to develop your own life, and, for a while at least, that life is with single women."

The other women in the group who are divorced or widowed murmur in agreement. These are all women who started out in their late teens or early twenties on the prescribed path for a Texas woman: marry early, marry up, and hang on to your husband's high status for dear life.

Stripped of her role as the beautiful accessory of a prominent man, what was left of Darlene was a 45-year-old woman without a college education who had to start over to complete the undone developmental tasks of her First Adulthood.

Her first priority was to catch up on the education she had missed as a child bride, but it had to provide more than a diploma. She needed something meaningful to do. By trial and error, she found she liked the medical field and built a rewarding career working with Alzheimer's patients in a nonprofit health care facility—a world formerly outside her experience. She also built the confidence that she could take care of herself financially.

All the while, however, she was going through a grieving process not unlike that of her widowed women friends. But like so many other women I interviewed, Darlene made a fascinating discovery, one that is closer to the secret of eternal youth than anything the drug companies are pushing. To repeat:

Sex and a passionate life go together.

Darlene wrestled with a social and religious environment that cast a single older woman who dated around as a hussy. "But I needed to regain confidence in myself as a sensual woman." She read a stack of self-help books and finally burned them all. When she dared to try dating, she was racked with guilt.

"Most of my religious friends dropped me. I just kept putting myself out there, trying different relationships and sexual encounters. I was so judgmental of myself—'This is wrong, I shouldn't be doing this'— because I was still coming out of a religious environment. So I set standards for myself: I should only sleep with one man at a time, and it had to be a committed relationship. But over the last eleven years, those 'shoulds' changed, as my sexual confidence has changed." She pauses. The other women want to hear more.

"Okay, I will admit that I have gone to bed knowing that there wouldn't be a committed, long-term companionship with a man." As her prudishness subsided, she developed a new personal code: "If the man is right and the mood is right, and he wants to and I want to, and I cause no harm to myself or to another, then it's okay for me." Darlene tucks one tanned leg tightly under the other and confesses, "Sometimes I feel like a *man.*"

Even in telling her story and receiving the group's affirmation, Darlene grows more radiant and declaratory. "Okay, I'm a fifty-six-year-old woman, I have a little tummy and cellulite, but my mental state now is so confident that anyone that I'm with is lucky to be with me. I'm awesome, look at this body!" She lifts out of her chair and does a little shimmy. "This is pretty cute!" We all laugh appreciatively. "I know how to flirt now, full force or just a little bit—whatever is necessary. Flirting is fun! I've come of age. I know who Darlene is. It's been a wonderful journey just to come out and be who I am."

After that spirited statement of independence, I thought I could guess the answer to my next question. "How do you feel about getting remarried now?"

Darlene tilts her head and surveys the group coyly. "I got married Friday."

Gasps, whoops, giggles, the room explodes.

"Well, who?"

"Who is it?"

"Who'd you marry?"

When Darlene drops the name "Wilson," there are more cheers. He is a man she met in her hiking group and has been dating off and on for ten years.

"Where's your ring?" is the next question.

"I took it off because I was afraid I'd be *X*'d out of the discussion group," she confesses, glancing at me. "Wilson adores me, there's passion, you've gotta have someone with energy and he's got it." She takes the blame for all their breakups but admits, "I've always tried to make him think they were his fault, to this day." She laughs. "I've dated and dated, I've looked under a lot of rocks, kissed a lot of frogs. Last January, Wilson and I started dating again, but now, at fifty-six, I'm ready to be married. I've crossed over that bridge. I want the companionship. I want to be able to pick up an ongoing conversation where it leaves off."

Darlene's midlife revolution is psychological, physical, and sexual. She has rebuilt her identity, her self-respect, her body, and her sexual élan. She found a new dream in working with Alzheimer's patients. And after more than ten years of being a Seeker and kissing a lot of frogs, she was passionate about her remarriage, a very different form of passion from what pushed her into her first marriage.

Boomer women like Darlene, although they grew up in the early giddy years of the sexual revolution, mostly missed out on it the first time around. They had already made their bed, since American women in 1960 married at an average age of 20 (by 2000, the median age of women's first marriage was 25). The Pill wasn't in widespread use until 1973, when 10 million women were using it as their main form of birth control. And as many of the women in the Fort Worth group agreed, in their day there had been two main reasons for hungering to get married as soon as possible.

"People got married at nineteen or twenty either because they were pregnant or because they wanted to have sex. In either case, you just had to be married."

As a result, many early boomer women followed the conventional path, marrying in their late teens or early twenties and becoming locked in early to the identity of caregiver in *his* world. Then along came the early-feminist perspective of the 1970s to challenge their choices. They have been living with that conflict all of their adult lives. Most attempted to make the traditional model of marriage and family work by trying harder and harder. But so often it blew up in a woman's face, no matter which way she went. I encountered many scenarios such as these:

Once the children are grown, she ascends to the level of her natural capacities and attains some recognition. More and more women of seasoned age are extending their education or developing long-deferred artistic ambitions. These are all esteem-building activities that allow a greater leap of growth. All of a sudden her husband begins sniping because he is no longer the only star in the house. Or she discovers on their AmEx invoice a charge for a Bermuda trip—for two.

From what I heard in interviews, men who married women in these generations are similarly conflicted. The man who married Holly the Helpmeet, whose role was to raise his children and help him advance his career, and who then later watches her late blooming as a community leader or brilliant businesswoman, might find himself falling head over dishwasher for his non-English-speaking maid, as does the Adam Sandler character in the 2004 movie *Spanglish.* Or for his assistant, personal trainer, or the cute little clerk in his accountant's office who writes his checks—any woman who looks up reverently to an older, wiser, wealthier man.

The man who married the plain Jane who later slides into a gray-haired, grandmotherly, bossy middle age may need a helium-pumped sexual fantasy to validate his continuing sexual prowess. He might well become addicted to Internet porn or be entranced by any one of the young single succulents swaying down the street or office corridors in their itty-bitty tanks and low-slung jeans with tattoos on their indentations as obvious as directional signals. Of course, many men do not fit these stereotypes. But it does require considerable resistance for both men and women in long-term marriages to bypass the many hazards of a sexually obsessed society such as ours.

A Religious Revolution

The Texas women are already on their second refill of coffee, we have been talking for more than an hour, and six of the eight women have yet to speak. This is going to be a deep-dish discussion!

Carol H. introduces herself with rueful amusement as a "recovering Christian fundamentalist." Carol is 53 and divorced, a striking woman, reed slim, sexy and graceful with green eyes, silver hair, and long tanned arms dangling from her sleeveless silk turtleneck. She wears cool cargo pants and sandals. One would not guess from the confidence she now projects that Carol was laid low by her divorce. In Fort Worth, she reminds us, "Not only do you lose a husband and your way of life, but your married friends turn away. All the support is gone in one fell swoop, and you're lying on the floor, you can't get up, and there's nobody to call because, down here, they shoot their wounded."

Her only refuge was the evangelical Christian church, where she was still accepted. It wasn't quite as rigid as the "cram-it-down-your-throat Christian church" in which she grew up. She had a brainstorm: Why not start a singles' group?

She had to fight church elders "who were fearful of anything new and certain that we were having sex on every outing." Her group lasted only two seasons, which the members thoroughly enjoyed, before the church was ripped apart by its own rigidity. Carol reexamined the religious "authorities" she had formerly accepted as the morality police and came to her own conclusion: "Whether it's the Jimmy Swaggarts or the Rush Limbaughs, Jerry Falwells or Bill O'Reillys, and most of the male religious conservatives, they're trying to control their own addictive sexual urges by trying to control women, but it never works for long."

Carol had already developed a new vocation as a psychotherapist, which gave her life meaning and helped her to view even times of difficult transition as opportunities for growth. "Anytime I've had a major emotional trauma," she says, "it has always, in the end, shifted me in terms of consciousness. So although it may be a really painful passage, it turns out in retrospect to have been wonderful."

Once she moved beyond the limited perceptions of fundamentalism, she says, she set off on a more internal spiritual journey. "All my life I'd heard the rubric 'The kingdom of Heaven is within,' but nobody knows what that means." Carol spent a good ten years of internal exploration— and this was after seeking therapy and joining Al-Anon. By reading and contemplating, she felt her consciousness change and expand. "I no longer needed that external validation. Deepak Chopra talks about seven levels of spirituality. Some people stay in third grade forever, some move on to sixth and seventh grade and graduate. You can apply that to many aspects of life, including relationships and sex."

Once a woman withdraws from her safe and familiar box and risks serious spiritual exploration, serendipitous things can happen. All of a sudden a life coach might appear in her backyard. It happened to Carol when she learned that a writer who had inspired her, Caroline Myss, a pioneer in the field of energy medicine and author of *Anatomy of the Spirit,* would be giving a small-group workshop in Mexico. Carol attended for a week. Being with like-minded Seekers was an intense and life-changing experience for her: "I walked through being alone, faced it, and found myself."

Carol now has more supportive friends and dates different kinds of men. Rather than the conventional three-piece-suiters who used to attract her, she gravitates toward men who are more open-minded, more spiritually conscious, more in touch with their creative side.

"It's getting harder and harder," she acknowledges. "There are plenty of men available, that's not the problem. I just don't think there are many of them in Fort Worth who are very conscious. They haven't worked much on themselves. It might be a lot easier in Sedona or Santa Fe. I'm challenged to find people who are like-minded, who actually care about the environment. Being able to have a deep and warm and exciting conversation is, to me, the aspect of any relationship that I value the most, whether it's with a man or woman."

Switching Off

There are many women who, having endured a painful divorce, have sworn off sexual involvements. Instead, they intensify their friendships and familial connections and often concentrate on their careers. According to Jean Giles-Sims, the sociology professor in the group, some of the female academics she knows distance themselves from dating or singles' groups, finding it difficult to attract men who think the way they do and being extremely committed to their work.

Judy Alter is a classic example. The only member of the Fort Worth group who isn't looking to date or mate again, Judy is in her mid-sixties. With her boy-cut gray hair and a roomy blouse over loose linen pants, she seems to be entirely comfortable appearing middle-aged. A true Texas woman who writes books and magazine articles and directs the academic press at TCU, Judy is bright and articulate and has been divorced for a long time. She indicates on her questionnaire that she is less interested in sex at 66 than she was at 56, describing herself as "wishful but too shy" to seek a partner.

When her turn comes in our discussion, she tells the group that after a rebellious marriage to a doctor, who then left her, she is not willing to take a chance again. She noticed a lowered libido after menopause, like many of the LLs among my respondents. Judy's adaptation has been to give up on sex. "I'm the mother of four and grandmother of three and they fill my life—not that I'm dependent on them, but they provide a lot of the love and companionship that I don't now have in a marriage." For safe social contact and to get out of the house, she cashiers on Saturday nights in a restaurant owned by friends. "They pay me in wine and steak." Primarily, Judy concentrates on her work, which is absorbing and creative. She was recently given a lifetime achievement award from the Western Writers of America. "I'm not sure that would have happened if I were focused on relationships with men."

These women powerfully demonstrate that even those who pursue a conventional path in their First Adulthood can find many different routes to turn off the beaten path in their Second Adulthood. Those routes can take them through a religious/spiritual revolution, like Carol; or an emotional/psychological/sexual revolution, like the newly remarried Darlene; or a deemphasis on sexuality and a deeper commitment to their work, like Judy.

But what about a woman who doesn't choose to make a revolution—isn't it possible to find a new self through evolution?

Chapter 8

The Spiritual Path

"*Y*ou don't have to be divorced to evolve."

It was several hours into the boisterous group discussion in Fort Worth when that statement, delivered with quiet conviction, startled us all. Heads turned toward Sandy McCall, the silver-haired psychotherapist, who describes herself modestly as "a small-town woman with red-state values, a marriage of almost forty years, two grandkids, and a sex life that is still extremely satisfying, though probably not as often."

All the while Sandy had been listening to the group of Texas divorcées and widows tell their stories, she had been thinking to herself that their situations were just like what she had lived through. "In midlife, I guess, we all become aware of some dimension that isn't fulfilled. It sounds like most of you needed to be freed sexually." The other women nodded. "I think all women in their forties or fifties come to a choice," Sandy continued. "Either they go back into a hole, or they're set free. But mine was not a sexual revolution. My revolution came from a desire of the spirit to be set free." She paused to gather her thoughts and spontaneously blurted out a strong religious metaphor: "Mine was a death and resurrection."

Startled intakes of breath were audible around the circle of women. How refreshing! In a society where most of us go for the quick fix, where a personal revolution may be seen as easier than working through a slow and sometimes painful evolution, Sandy's was a story we needed to hear. How does one precipitate enough change within the capsule of an existing marriage—break it open and reinvent it—to allow for a new level of mutual respect in both partners?

Sandy prefaced her story with the wise observation that all marriages go through cycles. "You may reach a point where you are disappointed, even despairing." The crossroads then points either to resignation and chronic resentment or to the risk of shaking up the relationship and insisting upon change. Sandy was able to summon the courage to accept the possible dissolution of her marriage unless there was a major change in her and her husband's unspoken contract.

The Midlife Power Struggle

Early marriage walled her off from the love beads, the crash pads, and the pot-juiced, rock-swooning collective sex party of the Sixties. Sandy started off like millions of women in the early to mid-Sixties, a whisker away from liberation by the Pill but longing for what comes next after heavy petting. In that era and before, nobody asked a woman what she wanted to do. It was assumed she would want what her husband wanted. In Sandy's case, Ron, the man she married in 1967, wanted her to support his dream of becoming a doctor. She taught school to support him through med school, until she got pregnant. Then, for the next fifteen years, their life together skidded around their four children like an endless circling of the skating pond, with less and less emotional warmth between husband and wife. Sandy's restlessness didn't surface until her late thirties. "I began to wonder, 'What do I want to be when I grow up?' " By her early forties, the restlessness had churned up layers of frustration.

"It was your midlife thing," she says, giving me a knowing smile. "When you get married, you make an unwritten contract. Our contract began during those med school years—to support him through his years of training and then work to pay off all the loans. When you get into the midlife stage, one or the other resents the contract and wants to change it or break it."

Sandy was so right. Dissatisfaction with the original marriage "contract" is entirely predictable in the passage to midlife. One partner is usually first to recognize the need to change the terms and conditions. If it is the wife, she is probably trying to make a first step into the more equitable power balance appropriate to a mature marriage. If the husband is still wedded to his role as the Strong One and expects her to continue in the role of his subordinate, he will feel betrayed and may retaliate.

The balance of the relationship is upset. This is to be expected.

"I was the dissatisfied one," Sandy tells our group. "I kinda thought it was my turn. We tried counseling but he just didn't hear me." Exactly what kind of change she wanted was not clear even to her. "I wanted more" is her classical answer. "More closeness. Intimacy." But pressed on this point by others in the group, Sandy raises a very different aspect of the contract that also needed revision: "I wanted more freedom, more equality, financial independence." This might sound like a contradiction, but, as many couples have found, freedom is actually the precursor to the mutual respect and closeness of a truly seasoned marriage. "The relationship had started out with him having the upper hand," Sandy continues. "I wanted to be heard. I don't know how to explain it . . . he wanted me to be one way, but I couldn't mold myself any further. I'm not sure it was only him, I probably thought I should be one way, too. But I was bending so far, I was breaking. My relationship with my husband was coming apart, it was heading towards divorce."

A classical dilemma for the traditional caregiving woman in early midlife: How to break out of the old pattern and find a new self without breaking up her family?

The paradox of love begins in the dueling impulses of our inner life. One impulse is to merge, surrender, and remain attached to a stronger person who will anticipate and meet all our needs and love us unconditionally; to restore, in some measure, the beatific closeness with Mother. The opposing impulse is to seek independence, to be separate, individual, to explore our capacities and become masters of our own destiny. The two urges are as competitive as two sports teams, which could be said to be managed by our Merger Self and our Seeker Self. This competition probably never ceases to play a part in our emotional life.

Throughout life, we have to keep rebalancing our need for intimate connection with our need for individuality. It is entirely predictable that the balance will be upset as we approach midlife. There is sure to be a struggle within—our inner dialogue can become as self-absorbed as it was in adolescence—but the tension will almost certainly play out for a long-married couple in the delicate arena of intimacy.

In Sandy's marriage, sex was not the problem. She and her husband had always enjoyed a robust sex life, at least in terms of frequency and the ease with which each could climax. But like so many women, as time went on, Sandy felt a painful breach between their physical connection and the emotional closeness for which she longed and that many men withhold, often without recognizing it.

She went back to school to get her master's degree, an idea her husband did not oppose so long as she continued to play her part in the tableau of a conventional marriage, acting as the supporting beam beneath the stage on which Ron starred as the indispensable, always-busy, always-a-pager-away, socially prominent cardiologist. But gaining a master's degree and the professional credentials to take on clients as a psychotherapist and help other people work through *their* problems—a rather typical solution sought by women in midlife who are stuck and foraging for their own salvation—did not change the pattern now well etched into her marriage.

Breaking up appeared to be the only way for Sandy to break out. But first she began to explore her suspended religious faith, attending the conservative Christian church in town that was growing by leaps and bounds. The evangelical promise reached her in a place that had long been empty. She did a great deal of soul-searching. The path that opened up the promise of a new life for her turned out to be a reconciliation with God. Once she began defining her values and her core self outside the realm of her marriage, her self-confidence began to build.

Ron could not relate to what Sandy called her "faith walk." He criticized her for being too soft, not tough enough for the real world.

"Weak. He thought I was weak." Her normally soft blue eyes flicker with anger. "I really think there's an awful lot of people like me," Sandy says. "Quiet, small-town people with traditional values who work hard and do the best we can. But a lot of the interactions in our marriage had been parent-child. When one person breaks that pattern, it upsets the balance. I was ready for adult-to-adult contact."

Sex was their only remaining connection, besides their children. "I think we both knew at an unconscious level that when the sex stopped, that would be the end," Sandy says. Their arguments were becoming more bitter, repetitive, exhausting. Her dreams were feverish. His dreams awakened him, sometimes with a strangled cry. They were both grieving. "Did somebody die?" she gasped on startling out of sleep one night. "Yes," she thought. It was their marriage, going through its death throes.

A Necessary Imbalance

As a couple enters midlife, usually beginning in the mid-forties, each partner may begin to resent being depended upon as a substitute parent by the other, and at the same time fear the accumulating evidence that she or he is, in fact, alone. No one can ever keep her safe. Or him.

It comes as a rude shock when the father-husband no longer wants to play the role of omnipotent protector, or when the child-wife grows up and talks back. Or when the reverse happens: suddenly he resents being "mothered" and feels smothered, or she gets fed up with being the only "adult" in the family.

Love is never free of the struggle over balance of power. And love always oscillates as the power balance changes, as observed by Dr. Ethel Person, professor of clinical psychiatry at Columbia University and a major contributor to the psychiatric literature on love and power. In her recent book *Feeling Strong,* Dr. Person writes, "People expect to find stability when they marry; they would do better to expect change—especially in the balance of power. Change can come so rapidly that one half of a couple becomes rudderless—or, rather, leaderless—at least until he or she is able to establish personal power."

One partner may declare an ultimatum: either things must change, or this relationship will be over. That can be a very healthy prod to a period of self-assessment for both partners, as it was for Sandy and her husband. It may be impossible to reconcile the tensions between the two partners' new aspirations. But it is also entirely possible that, given some space and time, they can reconnect on a different and deeper level.

"The way I looked at it," Sandy continues, "we'd built our house on sand, shifting sand, not on a rock, and it was crumbling. I felt like we had to get underneath the foundation with jackhammers and break it up and start all over." She was no longer going to surrender to her husband's control. But she yearned to merge with another source of love and safety.

Sandy found her path through spiritual revitalization. She replaced the faith she had attached to her successful husband—that he would always guide and care for her and love her unconditionally—with faith in a higher power. God would be her guide and provider of unconditional love. "The greatest proclivity to submission is in religious devotion," observes Dr. Person. Sandy lashed herself to her faith and hung on for dear life. It gave her the confidence to allow her marriage to go through a little death.

The McCalls agreed to an open-ended trial separation. Ron would move out to their weekend house. Each would pursue counseling on his or her own. At some point they would get back together and see if they "meshed."

As he was leaving, Ron turned, suddenly, almost lovably, a little lost. "Who will I talk to?" he asked.

"Talk to some of your friends."

"What friends? I don't have any friends I can really talk to."

"Well, figure out how to make some."

Easy enough for a woman to say; women cannot survive without friends to confess to, concoct fantasies of revenge with, soothe with bromides and shared self-help books; while men, particularly men in controlling professions, such as medicine, commonly arrive at midlife without a single friend who could be called a confidant—except the wife. And when the wife turns against them, they flounder.

Within days of their separation, Sandy was on the phone complaining about the car breaking down. "Who do I take it to?"

Her husband gave her back some of her own medicine. "That's your problem. Figure it out."

With some chagrin, Sandy realized that they had fallen into the same old well-worn grooves that had divided their parents' marriages. Her husband had depended totally on her to make friends and create their social life, and she had tendered to him all the practical aspects: the cars, their finances. "We'd divided responsibilities along traditional lines—we were actually keeping each other out of our domains," she observes. The other women murmur their recognition.

Five months into their separation, Sandy and Ron were resigned to the near certainty of divorce. They met with a mediator to discuss dividing their property. Sandy went from there on a silent retreat with her church. Whether by coincidence or because she was breaking inside, she ruptured a disc in her back, went home, and took to her bed. One night her husband asked to stop by and bring her dinner. No sooner had he fixed a tray than he said he had to go. "Oh," the disappointment leaked out of her voice. "I thought you were going to spend the evening with me."

He must have picked up on the fissure in her newfound self-confidence. "I've begun calling up some old friends, as you advised," he said proudly, "and they all tell me the same thing: she needs to know what it's going to be like without you, how tough it's going to be."

The composed response that came out of Sandy arose from her core. "Then they must not understand our relationship," she said, "because I know what it's like to be without you. I don't have a clue what it's like to be *with* you."

The truth of it pierced the atmosphere between them like a well-aimed dart. From that moment on, the disruption in the old balance began to be different, interesting, yeasty.

Her husband started insisting that he needed to move back in so she could see how he had changed. She said she didn't see much evidence yet. How could she see if he wasn't in her life? he asked. They went around that circular argument for a while, until Ron asked Sandy what she'd be willing to do.

"I know I've closed myself down, and you have too," she said. "I'd be willing to open my heart a little, to see if you've changed. Maybe we should just go out together on a date and get to know each other again."

A brilliant compromise.

She took pleasure in dressing for their date. He picked her up. The first time, he selected the restaurant, she the next. They didn't talk about their grievances. They talked about the things newly dating couples talk about—movies, books, what they like, who they are, and would you care for another glass of wine? When he drove her home and walked her to the door, he reached in front to turn the knob. She laid her hand gently on his.

"No. I don't do that on first dates." Truth was, she felt a little turned on herself, but she wasn't about to pop into bed and let him think everything was all right.

After the second date, he called. "That went well, don't you think?" Taking care to use a gently honest tone, Sandy said, "It was pleasant, yes. But if I was trying to get my wife back, I think I'd have gotten coverage and not taken calls from the hospital."

On a later date, Ron told her their separation felt like "a wound to the heart" and he wanted to try to re-create the laughter and fun they'd had early in their marriage. They agreed that before their next dinner date, they would each make a list of their needs and wants.

In the meantime, Ron was thrown by a staff crisis. His secretary of many years announced that she was taking another job. He didn't even know how to start the computer. Sandy offered to go into the office and help out. She took the opportunity to gain free computer training and administrative skills from the secretary. After a month's training, she found she liked her newfound power and stayed on, working part-time in his office. She and Ron had been a team when both were working toward his medical degree, but this was different. She gained more equality in the relationship by mastering the keeping of books. Meanwhile, her new vocation as a counselor was becoming a passion. She was also feeling secure for the first time that she could support herself. And she was learning how to be alone—astonished at all the things she could do on her own.

But Sandy's wants were not to be satisfied by more hugs or compliments on the home cooking her husband missed. The truth is, a woman can complain ad nauseam that her husband doesn't appreciate who she really is. But no major change in her partner's attitude can be expected until she finds out *for herself* who she wants to become, and sees and projects herself differently. Only then is it possible to know whether or not he can love and live with and, yes, measure up to this more evolved life partner.

Sandy's deepest desire was to know that she was loved by her Maker for the person He had made, and to reflect God's love in all her relationships. She told her husband, "I like finding out who I really am. If you can love this person that God created, fine. If you can't, maybe we can't be together."

Sandy's husband could see that the woman he had once known as his wife was, in reality, becoming reborn. He agreed to take a few steps on her faith walk. They began to discuss how, as part of the "new contract," they might rebuild the marriage on a faith foundation that was bigger than the two of them.

Laughter began to flow, unforced. He invited her to spend Fourth of July weekend at the weekend house with him. He warned her that he was on call at the hospital and he couldn't change it. She said, "Okay, I'll compromise, I'll bring my own car so I can leave when your beeper goes off and I won't get stuck." She went. He got no calls. She suspected he had bribed someone and gotten coverage. They didn't talk about going to bed together. It just happened. Under moonlight. Unbelievably exciting. She stayed overnight.

After a couple of months of dating, they took a long weekend trip together to Santa Fe, to see if they could enjoy each other again the way they had before. They took hikes and picked out the best restaurants and talked. For the first time, he agreed to go to the opera with her, and he seemed to enjoy it. For the first time, she relented on going for a balloon ride with him and, surprisingly, found the lighting of the flame exciting. The only time she got scared was when the balloon stopped moving and sat on a thermal.

Sandy cried out, "What if we fall right out of the sky?" She answered herself with a flippant serenity, "Oh, well, our kids are grown, what difference does it make?"

Knitting Back Together

Sandy was in her mid-forties when she set off on her midlife passage, began studying for her master's degree, and provoked the renegotiation in her marriage. She is 59 now and looking forward to more serenity in her sixties. When Sandy invited me to sleep over in the emptied bedroom of one of her grown children, the evidence of her reawakening abounded. She had created an office aerie above the stairs, where a psychotherapist's diagnostic manual lay open on the desk. The Post-it hung over her computer read, "Good morning. This is God. I will be handling all of your problems today."

Ron was the one who got up early and made breakfast for me. He lingered before going to work until Sandy awoke and gave him a kiss goodbye. Their home exuded comfort and an unforced elegance. Sandy told me she was looking forward to her sixtieth birthday in a few months. She and Ron planned to spend it in the mountain retreat they had built together, probably ungainly in purely architectural terms but set on rock as solid as the foundation on which their marriage had been rebuilt.

The couple has knitted back together in a far more important way. Not only has Ron become accepting of Sandy's spiritual search, they have found it meaningful to pray together. Eventually, they found a new church that resonates with both of them, and they attend together. "Part of the new contract was rebuilding the marriage on a faith foundation that is bigger than us," Sandy says. Finding a basis for a faith they can share has been enormously important in allowing them to move on to a true and lasting love.

What did she want to do in the next bonus decades? She enumerated some dreams for the near future: "I want to learn to speak French. I want to write a children's book. I want Ron, as he starts working less, to go on some mission trips with me, but also experience trips, like being the sailors on one of those old Nantucket freighters and rafting in the Grand Canyon—fun things. Hopefully, we'll still be able to do some exciting physical things into our seventies."

Sandy and her marriage had clearly evolved, but it had been a slow, spiritually guided evolution. She had come to an acceptance of who she is and what she most values and found, to her surprise, that her husband has come around to honoring, even revering, her for that authenticity.

"I woke up in the night and remembered the most important thing I wanted to clarify," she told me the next morning. "I have taught school, I've been a therapist, I've facilitated training seminars, I've done public speaking, what else? Oh, yes, I've been an educator on drug and alcohol abuse and done marketing seminars, and I write for magazines. They were all well and good, and I enjoyed them a lot. And I still do some of them, but I like who and where I am now.

"You asked me what I wanted to do. I realize that the most important thing in the world to me is being a wife and mother, and now a grandmother—it's the best! It's the only thing I've found that is not over-rated.

"What I really hope is that somewhere within my sphere of influence I can touch people's lives with an act of kindness, a word of wisdom, a healing touch. The only way I know how to do that is to be present in the place where I have been planted. And that is being a wife, mother, grand-mother, and friend. I think how blessed I am to live in a free country where I have the opportunity to touch people's lives and be touched by those who come in my path."

When we turned to more lighthearted subjects, Sandy asked if I had seen her favorite movie, *The Notebook*. I had, and I'd found it deeply moving. It is the story of an intense young love, thwarted by disapproving parents and only tragically revived when the woman is elderly and in-stitutionalized, sinking into the fog of Alzheimer's disease. Her former lover, played as an older man by James Garner, finds her and visits every day to read to her from a notebook where he recorded the saga of their intense romance and forced separation. The woman, played by Gena Rowlands, is eventually drawn out of her fog by his indefatigable efforts to revive the memory of their great love. They share a brief but ineffably tender reconnection. And when he learns that she is about to die, he joins her in her institutional bed and they pass on together.

For Sandy, the movie evoked the image of her husband's parents, who underwent a radical change in their late eighties. "I never saw him touch his wife or heard him tell her he loved her," she says. "But now they're living together in an assisted-living home. They've pushed their beds together and he gazes at her—this eighty-nine-year-old man—and says, with great enthusiasm, 'I *love* this woman!' They have come full cir-cle. To me, the whole purpose of life is to come full circle."

Chapter 9

Sagas of *Un*seasoned
Men and Women

*H*e is a 63-year-old bachelor who is still sexy and charming enough to romance only women under 30. Having recently sold his hugely successful hip-hop record company, he is flush and free to loaf around Tahiti or jet to Paris for dinner. This night, after much champagne, he is standing on the Pont Neuf looking down at the Seine as a party barge passes beneath him, and he catches the strains of a balladeer singing "La Vie en Rose."

Why is this man crying his eyes out?

He has just been jilted by a woman who taught him for the first time what love is all about. She is accomplished, brainy, quirky, and very attractive—that is, if a man can get past the fact that she is middle-aged and postmenopausal, colors her hair, and wears turtlenecks in summer. He didn't get past those externals until it was too late. The woman he loves—a woman of 55—has been swept away by a drop-dead handsome doctor in his early thirties. She dumped our aging bachelor for a younger lover.

The bachelor stands on the bridge in Paris dripping tears and mocking himself: "Look who gets to be the girl."

      *   *   *

It is commonly assumed that males in midlife are the ones who do the dumping—although now we know it's women who are initiating most of the after-45 separations. It is also assumed that men have a much easier time replacing the women in their lives—they certainly do it a lot sooner than divorced or widowed women. Psychiatrist and author Irvin Yalom, having seen many widowed men in his lengthy practice, laments, "Men re-pair so fast, they often don't have time to repair themselves."

Not so fast anymore. The above character, played by Jack Nicholson in *Something's Gotta Give,* is not an aberration. Many men in their late fifties and sixties tell me that the world has turned upside down. They can no longer be assured of being the ones who love and leave, even when the woman is close to their own age. *Especially* when the woman is close to their own age. She may turn the tables and dump *him* for a younger man. Or for the love of a woman. Or just to go out in the world and pursue her own passion.

"They won't commit" is the new complaint of pre-senior men. I hear it even from highly eligible divorced men with advanced degrees who have lots of time on their semiretired hands. They want the previous edition of woman, the one who will devote herself to them, arrange their lives, travel with them, be home waiting for them. But the women in their age group who are active and attractive may be too busy with their own still-expanding personal universes. An ever-smaller number are willing to give up their own stimulating work and sideline the friends, children, and grandchildren who sustain their lives with reliable joy, to act as the full-time organizer, travel agent, and nurse to an older, unreconstructed man.

Let's look more closely in this chapter at a few of the many unattached men and women over 50 who are out there, trying like mad to find dates, sex, love—even if it's just cyberlove—and having no luck. What can we learn from their mistakes?

Shopping for the Perfect 10

Men are not the only ones hobbled by unrealistic expectations in the singles' bazaar. In a group interview with women from the San Francisco Bay area I met Claudia, a cultivated Jewish woman of 53 with beautifully chiseled features, green eyes, a float of long dark hair. Her sexy body was suggested through a lacy black shirt and clingy pants. She is divorced and politically liberal, and she has had no luck whatsoever in attracting prospective dates online. Here are the highlights from Claudia's Match.com profile:

About me and who I'd like to meet:

> Smart, sexy, sophisticated, striking, slender, refined, educated, funny, attractive, charming, warm—opera, symphony, jazz, blues, cooking, singing, walking, working out, nature, theatre, ballet, travel, language, reading.

Claudia also notes in her profile that she has a graduate degree, speaks Russian, and earns more than $150,000 a year in an executive capacity. As if that list weren't enough to scare off lesser mortals, she is highly specific about what she wants:

About My Date

Height:	5'10"
Education:	Graduate Degree, PhD/Post Doctoral
Job:	Financial Services, Legal, Medical/Dental
Income:	$150,000+
Turn-Ons:	Flirting, Dancing, Power, Money, Brainiacs, Boldness/Candlelight, Thunderstorms

It sounds as if Claudia wants a mirror image of herself and she is interested only in a financial manager, lawyer, doctor, or dentist, seemingly the kinds of men of whom her mother would have approved. She tells us, "I haven't been out with one person, not one. I've e-mailed several men, back and forth, but if there's the slightest thing that I find that strikes me the wrong way, I'll just say, 'No, forget it.' "

One man sounded intriguing enough that she e-mailed back and forth with him, until he pushed her to meet in person. She kept putting him off with "I'd like to chat a little bit more online before we meet." He replied, "I don't have time for online chit chat."

Claudia e-mailed back: "I would at least like to know how you write, because that means a lot to me." She wanted to test his grammar and spelling and assure herself that he was up to her standards. He was offended.

"So we had an e-mail fight before we even talked on the phone!" says Claudia, laughing. She e-mailed him, "I don't think this is going to work out, I think you've got an edge."

He responded, "I'm a dry, sardonic New Yorker."

She replied, "Well, I'm not into dry and sardonic. I'm into sophisticated, intelligent, elegant, and polite."

That was the end of that pre-relationship.

In our conversation, Claudia revealed that her Match.com profile is a little out of date and not fully honest—a no-no in cyberdating. She is actually out of a job, though she did have a managerial position before being laid off. "I'm looking for a new avenue," she says. Her deepest emotional engagement is with her only child, a junior in high school. "My ex-husband is a very devoted father, and we both have been concerned with her well-being first and foremost." Claudia is busy ferrying her daughter around to look at colleges. She has not yet experienced the empty nest. And she is not yet serious about anticipating the next stage of her life.

CheckMates

A solution to Claudia's frustration with the online dating world might lie with Carole Shattil, founder of CheckMates Inc. and a Bay Area professional matchmaker for fifteen years. She has 2,500 men and women in her database whom she pairs up, calling on her training in psychology to decide who will meet whom. Her goal is to save her clients from themselves. The rise in online dating, she says, has caused an epidemic of fibbing and exaggeration. "I asked someone I was interviewing how old he was, and he said, 'Well, would you like my Internet age or my real age?' "

Weight and job status are two other rarely revealed truths. Carole's job is to weed out the blatant mistruths plaguing the majority of profiles on online matchmaking websites. "What I do is find people who would be good for each other and present them to one another." But Carole does more than that. She does background checks on her clients, sometimes contacting their places of business to be sure they work where they say they do. She examines their marital history, their hobbies, their personal goals, and their relationship wants and needs. She takes photos herself to make sure they are current.

The art of matchmaking, however, is not about throwing together two people who like to ski and hoping for the best. Carole often acts as a relationship coach. "The most successful men—I'm talking about Harvard and Yale—can be so naive about how women think and feel." Often recently divorced or widowed, many of the men haven't been on the dating scene in a long time and need some guidance.

"I had a conversation with a man the other day about the difference between real breasts and silicone breasts," Carole says. "When the man got married, there was only one kind; he just didn't know about silicone." She also emphasizes to her midlife female clients the importance of condoms. "Some of them obviously haven't dated since they were twenty years old. They're used to a long-term, monogamous relationship. They trusted their husbands. So when they go out there now, it's like another world for them."

If a match Carole sets up is not working out, she meets with the woman and man individually and takes down their complaints. Then she provides them each with feedback, and suggestions: X and Y didn't really work; next time you might try Z.

Midlife singles may have a lot in common with Claudia and her incredibly high expectations. "Everyone's much more particular as they get older," says Carole. "If they're going to put their energy into a relationship, they're going to want someone to be compatible with them sexually, physically, intellectually, and emotionally. They don't want to make the same mistake twice." CheckMates Inc. is particularly helpful for older, finicky, and unseasoned singles. Instead of shouting into cyberspace and hoping for perfection to come back, Carole can help a client tailor her expectations to reality and let her know when she, not her date, is the problem. But Carole won't stop looking until her clients are happy. "I had one woman who just wouldn't settle for less than a Ph.D. And he had to be within five miles of her." Tall order, right?

"No, she waited a good four, five months for the right person. We found him."

Men and women who have been divorced and seeking new partners for some years may still be holding on to unrealistic expectations of finding the perfect husband or the replacement wife. They may not know how to, or are afraid to, move on to the more egalitarian relationships that are possible in midlife and later. Let's meet some of these long-term Seekers and see what can be learned from them.

Mineola Men's Lotto

It's take-out spaghetti and meatballs at Dennis's place in Mineola on Long Island, New York. It's all men, gathered to gripe about last Saturday night's singles' dance, again a disaster.

Paul is the last to show up, looking handsome and sporty with tanned arms showing under his polo shirt and a full head of wavy gray-black hair. In his brusque business school manner, he unfolds what seems to be a racing sheet. The guys eagerly pass it around and check out the numbers Paul has circled. But he's not touting the ponies. He's touting the singles' events listed for the next week in the Long Island edition of *Newsday.* He has circled all those that sound interesting and have an admission fee under $18.

The five men who have gathered in Dennis's original Cape Cod house are all, as they are quick to say, "quality men." They all possess advanced degrees, are all trim for their age ("We eat small portions and avoid dessert—it makes us more marketable"), and all are eager for decent dates. Just about every weekend they try a dance or other singles' events. During the week they meet either at the local diner or in Dennis's kitchen. Only the menu changes; the conversation is usually the same.

"Could you believe it? Seventy men to thirty women at that last dance," complains Paul. At 59, he has been downsized from his job as a marketing executive and is now an independent sales consultant. "I went over to a table of six or seven women, all dressed to the nines, and said, 'Ladies, how can you expect a man to approach your pack? Doesn't any one of you want to break away from the herd and risk bumping into a guy?'"

The guys all agree that it's much easier to approach a single woman who's standing at the edge of the dance floor or alone at the bar, radiating "passion and confidence." Alan, a self-employed graphic designer with a warm, dimpled smile and a meaty handshake, has become quite strategic in his approach: "When I see one I like, I'll camp out by the ladies' room. It's only a matter of time."

The host, Dennis, a bookish-looking man with a long thin nose, deep-set eyes, and gray, wavy hair, broods, "You see the same obese women. They approach you, and when you're not interested, they seem annoyed. Don't they realize that the weight is the reason? But bring this up at a mixed singles' discussion group, and you'd better be very close to the door."

Dennis is particularly handicapped at the singles' dances because of his opening gambit: "I'm a numismatist."

"Huh?"

"I deal in rare coins."

"Can you even make a living at that?"

"I wrote a book about it," he states proudly. He might even offer to produce the handsomely illustrated tome, which he self-published and was well-received in his field. If he begins with this opening dialogue to nowhere, Dennis doesn't get to mention that he formerly worked for an elite Wall Street firm. He complains to his friends that women are always trying to find out whether a man is "financially secure" before they waste too much time talking to him. These men have read all the singles' guides. They've tried adult education classes, yoga classes, even taken ballroom dance lessons. "I haven't found the magic formula," admits Paul.

What kind of woman do the men find attractive? I ask.

"A beautiful blonde with a great body and who dresses well. You go from there to see if there's some chemistry and compatibility."

This is, of course, the stuff of fantasy—roughly equivalent to Diane Keaton meeting a baby doctor who looks like Keanu Reeves and having him tell her on their first date, "You're incredibly sexy." That's why we go to the movies.

After several years of trying, not one of the men has found this ideal partner, but their expectations have not diminished.

Tulsa Women's Two-Step

It's going to be another night at the Bobbiesox Club for Cindy, Sue, and Juanita, three smart, single nurses in Tulsa, Oklahoma. "We don't wear Manolo Blahniks like Sarah Jessica Parker, we wear boots or sandals, but we have our own little *Sex and the City* sort of life out here in the heartland," they assure me. Tulsa is a very different environment from Long Island, to be sure, but the women's hunger for decent dates equals that of the Mineola men.

The Bobbiesox Club is a karaoke club for locals who are divorced or widowed and who belong to a generation that loves getting behind a hand mike and pretending to be Elvis or Bette Midler. Sue and Juanita are seated on stools at a high table, sipping beer from mugs. Juanita describes their emotional ages: "Sue is our two-year-old. I'm the teenager. And Cindy is the grown-up. We support each other in the lives we have chosen." Ten years of single life have taught Juanita an indelible lesson: "Relationships with men come and go, but what sustains you are your girlfriends."

Cindy is late. She's driving two hours back from meeting yet another hopeful online dating contact. "This is where we come to play—it's recess," says Sue, dangling a backless sandal from the end of her long, slender leg. She is an outrageous flirt. When she gets finished working as an RN at a psychiatric hospital, she takes her time dressing up to go to one of the several karaoke clubs around town. She takes off her stiff white uniform and slithers into a long, floaty, translucent dance dress, blows out her tinted ginger hair, repaints her nails fire engine red, takes off her glasses, and outlines her eyes as precisely as she writes up a hospital chart.

"I am a work in progress, beginning a whole new life," Sue says. She is 51 and still chokes up when she talks about the husband she lost seven years ago. He left her well off with a big insurance policy. "But I was so angry at him for dying because he wouldn't take care of himself," she confesses, "I couldn't get rid of that money fast enough!" In the last year her house was repossessed, she was diagnosed as bipolar, and she has made a radical decision. "I always thought I needed a man in my life. But going to therapy and reading a lot of different philosophies, you know what? Maybe I don't need a full-time partner," she tells Juanita. "I like having four men in and out of my life."

Juanita, whose brunette locks are elaborately teased because she is not ready to give up her generation's claim to fame—big hair—shakes her head. "When did this decision happen?"

"Just the last couple of weeks," Sue blurts out.

Juanita, who was happily married for twenty years, recounts the epiphany she had at the age of 40. She and her sister had gone off to Galveston to comfort a recently divorced friend. One day, while the three women were reveling in their rare girl time and skinny dipping on the beach, Juanita burst out crying. "What I had found that weekend was a part of myself that I had lost—the one who was full of laughter and delight. I came back and told my husband, 'Something has to change here, and I'm not sure what it is.' " She begged him to go to a marriage counselor with her. He said, "I don't think we necessarily have to go over all that stuff from our past."

Over the next five years Juanita did a lot of therapy and read self-help books. One line stuck with her: "Do you want to be right? Or do you want to be happy?"

"I quit making him wrong and insisting that I was always right. After a heart-wrenching process, I let him go."

Juanita is sobered to realize that ten years have elapsed since her divorce. "I have an active life, tons of friends, but it hit me when I had my fiftieth birthday this year. I had just taken a big job—director of nursing at a psychiatric hospital. This is the first time an employer realized that I can do something and do it well. But I have nobody to go home to and share my day with."

Men at the club buzz around the two nurses; these are men they know and like to joke and dance with but whom they would never, ever, take home. A sixty-something man is particularly attentive to Sue. She confides, "He would have me in a minute if I would have him, but that man would just baby me and pamper me and pet me and there would be no challenge." Sue says the men who frequent clubs usually have more than one marriage behind them and they don't even know where all their kids are—they've lost touch. "And if they go out to clubs every night, they don't expand their minds. They can be bores."

Juanita admits, "I've had men tell me that I'm somewhat selfish. I tell them they may be right. But for years I gave all, and gave some more, and so I'm kind of proud of being selfish at this point."

Cindy arrives, looking pretty but pissed. She is all dressed up in her best black sheath, with ankle-strap sandals that show off her shapely, slender legs. Cindy is a milk-fed, heartland version of Mia Farrow, petite and blond with a soft, breathy voice. But the last ten years in the singles' scene have made her a good deal harder than she appears. And much pickier. Tonight didn't help.

Sue and Juanita pump her about the date.

"He had a yellow Porsche, he was nice-looking, I would have been attracted to him. We go into a very nice restaurant. But then I think I asked him one question, and he jumped right into how he hasn't paid taxes for thirteen years! According to him, the IRS set out to ruin him. So he found God and spent the past eight years reading the Bible—in Greek. He now makes a living, off the books, by teaching other people how to avoid paying their taxes. And this was worth a four-hour round-trip?"

Like Juanita, Cindy is shaken by the realization that she has now been single for a decade. "When I first went out on the singles' scene, if I heard anybody say they had been single for more than five years, I would think, 'There must be something really wrong with that person.' " But here she is, after trying out seven different dating sites and many different men, still finishing off the night at the Bobbiesox with her girlfriends.

Cindy is a congenital nurturer. As a neonatal nurse, she cares for other people's sick babies and premature infants. But after a life spent ensuring the happiness of those around her, Cindy is now looking out for number one. In her peevish mood, she snaps, "I've given up trying to find someone that I can dance with and sleep with and have a decent churchgoing relationship with—they just don't exist!"

Men Looking for TLC

Back in Mineola, Dennis is in a pensive mood. "It used to be the men were the ones you had to drag into the relationships," he says. "Now the women don't need us, for families or for money. They're self-sufficient, and they're calling the shots. Women have always called the sexual shots, and now that they're making enough money, they have the financial advantage. What does that leave us with? There's been a role reversal."

Dennis is a worrier, sweet-natured but obsessively detailed. "I live alone, I work alone," he says. "I wake up at four o'clock in the morning—it happens a lot—feeling like 'Here I am again, another night alone in this bed.' What brought me into the singles' scene was, I was in a relationship with a woman for thirteen years, from the time I was forty-two to fifty-five," he tells us. "When that broke up, I had no idea about what to do, it had felt to me like a marriage. All of a sudden, wow, it was like somebody dropped a fifty-pound weight on my head. The women had changed in those thirteen, fourteen years," from the end of the 1980s into the 1990s. "It is a whole different world now, turned upside down. I feel like now *we* are the women."

The other men nod in sober recognition.

"I had a wonderful wife for twenty years," says Paul. "She was a 10. I lost her to heart disease. I don't want to settle for second best, for an average woman who's a 5 or even a 7.5. You say to yourself in every relationship, 'What am I getting out of this?' I did have true feelings for a beautiful blond doctor. I took her back to her house, expecting coffee, and she led me into the bedroom. She took the lead. It was amazing. . . ." He rolls his eyes.

The guys murmur vicariously. They say they love it when a woman is confident enough to take the lead sexually.

Paul adds a regretful postscript: "But with the doctor, I realized her mother comes first or her job comes first. At the time I was seeing her, she was still legally married. And she was determined to have a baby. So I was the low man on the totem pole."

Throughout the evening, Paul insists that he's not going to settle for less than a 10. Of course, the image of his wife is frozen in time—she died in her mid-forties, and he never saw her aging. Any woman he compares to her will be up against impossible competition with a phantom.

"I'm not comparing women I meet to my wife," he contends.

"But you keep saying you're not going to settle for anything less than what you had. Isn't that a comparison?"

"I guess what I'm saying is that the physical appearance could be very different," he concedes. "I tend to date a lot of blondes now, and my wife was a brunette. I date women who are a little bit taller than she was—she was five foot three. I date women five-four to five-seven."

"You're really giving them a lot of rope," teases one of the guys.

Women Shopping for Gourmet Sex

The Tulsa nurses, like many women who become single after 40, have spent some years sampling the wares in the singles' supermarket and have become quite the connoisseurs of sensual pleasure. They are looking for love, too, of course, but they seem even more picky in the sexual department than some of the men I've interviewed.

"I didn't know how great sex could be," Cindy says, twirling her swizzle stick and grinning. "I thought that it was highly overrated, that it was a better thing for guys than for women. Now that I've had some different partners, I know how great it is and I don't want it episodically." She is not interested in one-night stands. "I feel I deserve a regular sex partner and the romance and closeness that go with it." She looks around the club and wrinkles up her nose. "Now I'm pickier, because I've learned that some guys kiss horribly, some guys don't like to be touched, they just go right for the kill, and some think they're studs when they're anything but. You cannot undo fifty years of their lovemaking habits. And I don't want to educate someone else."

Juanita is on early call at the hospital, but she scans the denizens of the Bobbiesox Club one more time before she goes home. "A lot of these guys would like to be with me, but they're flighty, not grounded. They want me to be the grounding. But what I tell the men I date is, I'm in charge all day in my day life. I don't want to be in charge in my night life."

Cindy is dead honest about why she winds up at the Bobbiesox Club more nights than she would like: "I go to clubs because it forces me to get out of my scrubs and get cleaned up. Dancing is a way to be held without being screwed."

The last online suitor who made her heart flutter was a man named Johnny. He wrote wonderfully sensitive e-mails. "He was a churchgoing man who was able to express higher thoughts," Cindy says. But whenever they got ready to meet in person, Johnny backed out. This is a ubiquitous complaint for both genders who seek romance online. Women tend to chicken out and push the "block button" when an Internet suitor becomes too eager to close the deal. Men have their own brutal style. They are more likely to show up for the first face-to-face meeting, glimpse the woman through the window of the café, and split.

Heavy of heart but angry at Johnny's ambivalence, Cindy finally gave up on her last Internet suitor. She informed him she would not accept any more of his e-mails.

One of the better dance partners approaches Cindy, and she is happy to float around the floor in his arms, enjoying the illusion of romance. "Dancing is the only time in our lives where we don't have to lead," she confides. "We have to lead sexually because we deal with a lot of wounded men. The men of our age are scared. Their wives left them, and their egos are shit—that's why they want to be with younger women. We want men to lead, in some way besides on the dance floor. We want occasionally to have a soft place to fall. I don't want to date just to boost somebody's ego! I'll meet them halfway, but I want somebody to boost *my* ego."

Singles: Your Own Worst Enemy

That's what Alan would call his book if he ever writes about his painful experiences starting his own singles' group on Long Island. "Singles are always using the word 'realistic,' but most aren't," he says. "They're too wrapped up in themselves." He acknowledges, "We all have expectations of meeting people on a certain educational level, economic level, and spiritual level—and within five to ten years of our own age." He picks out a letter from the stack of complaints he routinely receives, this one from a woman in her early forties who paid to come to a dance he advertised as "for midlife singles." The irate woman wrote, "Way too many of the men were over 50, some even looked like 60. That's way over what you advertised. Next time you should check people's IDs at the door for their real ages."

Alan chuckles in spite of himself. "Can you imagine being carded at a midlife singles' dance?"

Alan started the club five years ago hoping to create a network of friends, male and female. "If I don't do this, I'll sit home and eat Ben and Jerry's until I'm three hundred pounds."

Three of the five men gathered in Dennis's living room now "work from home." Like so many men in their age group of late fifties to early sixties, they no longer have full-time, salaried jobs. It is my observation, after interviewing a number of such men, that their self-image often deteriorates once they lose their professional identity. If they don't find a new dream, they can become their own biggest obstacle in finding a satisfactory new partner.

Alan departs significantly in attitude from the other men in the Mineola group. He is grateful about being single. He is one of the men represented in the AARP statistic about divorces after the age of 40; his wife initiated theirs, and he never saw it coming. "I went from my parents' house to a marital house, and I didn't know myself at all. Frankly, divorce was the best thing that happened to me—for personal growth. It's only since I've been in the singles' world that I've learned how to function on my own."

"The women all love Alan," says Paul enviously. Why? Alan is a listener. He has evolved into the kind of man who is invited on numerous "girls' nights out," learning from his female friends what he didn't know about marriage all the years he tried to play the role of husband. While Paul is looking for a woman who's a 10, Alan says he's looking for ten different women. "I've realized there are so many females in the world— they smell different, they feel different, they speak differently, they think differently. I am just so enamored, even in some relationships I have with women where there is no sex. I'm learning so much about life."

The Tulsa Backup Plan

Not one to sit around and bemoan the deficits in her life, Cindy always has to have a goal. Over the past few years she has pursued her passion for horses. Together with her ex-husband, she bought a piece of flat, unimproved land on a pretty creek and turned it into a fifteen-acre horse farm, complete with a barn and apartment. "This was my baby. I love it out there," she says with fervor, pulling out photos of her horses to show around. Her ex lives on the horse farm for now, while she and their daughters live in his house in town to be near their school districts. "He drops by the town house almost every day to pick up his mail and see the kids," she says, with pride in engineering this arrangement. "Occasionally, he runs into the men I'm going out with." With strong emphasis she adds, "As the father of my children, he will always be in my life."

After ten years of experimentation on the singles' scene, Cindy says she knows what she needs to know to have a sublime marriage—if only she could find the right life partner. She resists taking on another career or home improvement project, being committed to keeping herself free over the next few years to work on a relationship—if one seriously presents itself. "If I met the right man, I'd move to Timbuktu to be with him," she vows.

Behind that vow is a strong inner contradiction. Even as Cindy yearns to escape from her congenital habit of caring for everyone else and professes to want a strong emotional and sexual connection with a new man, she is still deeply attached to her first family. She is accustomed to exercising full maternal control over her children and is still very attached to her ex-husband. She likes being depended upon. She likes running the show.

Intelligently, however, Cindy has a backup idea all worked out: "If I don't marry, I've picked out a wonderful Oklahoma farmhouse with a huge porch, and my plan is—because you've always got to have a plan—my ex would sell the house in town and build a new house out on the farm. He and I would share the cost. Then I'd live on one side of the creek and he'd live in the apartment on the other side. And when our kids would come home, we'd have six bedrooms and our grandkids could sleep over with us. The alternative is, I meet a guy who can afford to build me the house. I have no problem with my ex living on the other side of the creek, if it wouldn't bother my new man. Anybody I meet has to realize how important my ex-husband is in my life."

It's all very neat, but here's the rub: men are territorial about their woman. Zoologically speaking, Cindy's stallion might accept a new male on the farm, but it's not likely that two human males could coexist on the same fifteen acres with only one mated to the female. Cindy has some insight into her unrealistic expectations: "A lot of men are threatened by my ex-husband being so much in my life. I also have five children and work nights every weekend. Maybe that's why I'm still single."

Half a Cake Is Better Than None

For all his complaining about the singles' scene, Dennis actually is the one man in the group who doesn't need to be out there: he has a girl-friend, an attractive woman considerably younger than he. But he knows he's not her be-all and end-all.

"She has a circle of friends she had developed before she met me who she likes to spend time with—girlfriends," he says, eyebrows arched in disbelief. "Also, she has three children; a son who lives with her, two married daughters, and grandchildren. She likes to divide her time among the grandchildren, her children, her girlfriends, and myself. So there are times where I feel that I am being put second or third." The ultimate mystification, he confides, was when his girlfriend announced that she wanted to go off to a spa for a weekend—by herself!

Paul jumps on this: "Hey, Dennis, she's controlling the situation. You have to look for somebody else. You're wasting your time. You've got to move on."

Dennis continues to plead his case: "I live alone, I work alone. She goes out in the field, she meets people with her job, whereas I'm more isolated. So I have, I guess, more of a need to expand the relationship." But his girlfriend has told him that she doesn't want to get married again. Baffled, he says, "I get the impression she doesn't even want to co-habitate."

I lay out the Tulsa nurses' point of view: "Women that we're talking about—the ones who don't want to get married, who put limitations on how much time they can give you, have other familial and personal interests, and they don't want to give up their girlfriends. They don't want to have to be with you 24/7. They want a more equitable deal."

Paul protests. "That's not the real world. For success in a good marriage, you have to be willing to make sacrifices for your partner. And I don't see women fully understanding that you must do that."

I point out the obvious: "Making sacrifices is what most of the women we're talking about feel they did for twenty or twenty-five years. Then either she got dumped, or he didn't grow and she did, or she soared in her career and he felt overshadowed, or he began drinking, or he got sick and she took care of him and he died anyway. Now the women say, 'If I have a multifaceted life, I'm not going to be devastated if a romance doesn't work out.' They don't expect of you what your first wife did: 'I need you to father my children, protect me, and take care of me financially.' They're not pushing you to the altar or putting you in the mortgage bind. They may even say that as long as you are honest with each other, you can both be dating more than one person. That kind of egalitarian balance is what many of us have said we've always wanted. But do guys really want that?"

"I want the whole ball of wax," says Paul unapologetically.

"You want what you had in your marriage," I prompt.

"Yes. I was happy before, why can't I be happy again? My wife was a nurturer, she was a mother, she was a homemaker, she raised my son, she took care of me and the house. She was brilliant financially; she took care of the checkbook. I did spend time with her. Vacations we planned together, we did renovations on the house together. What I find lacking in a lot of the women I meet is, they're not willing to take that risk of being a partner. There's something holding them back."

I suggest to Paul that he has just described the kind of partnership more appropriate to the child-rearing years. But at this later stage, women are looking more for a life partner. I did not point out to Paul that when he was "happy before," he brought a different package to the table. Then, he was rising in his career as a marketing executive, earning stock options and an income in a top tax bracket. Looking at it through his lens, *he* was a 10. Then. Five years ago his company tanked, his stock options were rendered worthless, the stock market crashed. He passed 55 and was downsized. Like many men whose careers have been narrowed by corporate ageism, Paul will never be a 10 again in those same narrow terms.

Just then Alan has an *Aha!* moment: "I never understood—till tonight, Paul—that you're still trying to get that marriage back. And as Gail says, women who are now in their forties and fifties, they've done that. So you may have to relax what you're looking for."

◆   ◆   ◆

Dennis has something special to offer the men tonight: he remembered that it is Paul's birthday. After the take-out spaghetti, he appears from the kitchen proudly bearing one half of a store-bought chocolate cake, covered in candles, and a bowl of strawberries. The men all laugh and applaud.

The confidences they are able to share, plus remembering a birthday, are some of the things that make Dennis's group a soul saver for these men. For men, perhaps the best part of the shift in gender characteristics that takes place in middle life is their need and willingness to form real friendships with other men. During their competitive years, men rarely dare to confide in one another. But once beyond the dog-eat-dog stage, they can let down their barriers, become more tolerant of their own and others' weaknesses, discuss their problems, hopes, and dreams, and offer one another support. In fact, scientific studies have shown that men who have four or more real friends in whom they can confide actually live longer.

The brightest side of midlife for women is the assertiveness that grows as they become seasoned. It's what allows the Tulsa nurses to tell men what they really think. It's what helps them to get up the nerve to meet face-to-face with yet another contact they make online.

An e-mail I recently received from Cindy, the neonatal nurse, proved the point. Johnny—the elusive e-mail suitor on whom she had given up—finally e-mailed and said he wanted to meet her. It turns out that he's a horse trainer who lives an hour away on twenty acres, a man who shares her passion. They have had two fun dates, and Cindy writes, "I don't believe I've ever been this comfortable with a person of the opposite sex. Don't know where it's going, but the ride is fun!"

Persistence pays. Although the men and women in this chapter have not yet found their key to becoming seasoned, that doesn't mean they will remain stuck. There is no clear map: this is uncharted territory. We are all just beginning to learn how it's done.

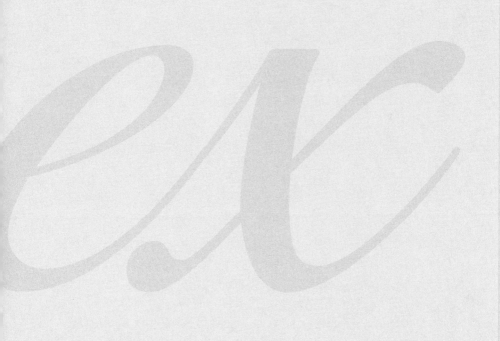

Part II

The Romantic Renaissance

*Y*ou're distracted. You forgot your meeting or misplaced your phone, but even the dark, rainy day is desperately romantic. Your feet soar as you hurry down the street to meet him. The music in the cafés seems written for you. Your heart's vibrating as constantly as the strings of a street-corner fiddler. The sexual buzz just beneath your skin is incessant. So saturated are you with wonder of new love that you see him everywhere. Is that him with his hand caressing the rump of another woman, the bastard? No, there he is disappearing into a cab—he's not going to wait! Your innards are tumbling, you start running, you trip off the curb. You're half crazy, but oh, isn't it sweet?

Remember those feelings? They are the harbinger of the Romantic Renaissance.

A seeker of the passionate life will go through a series of phases, usually beginning with the Romantic Renaissance. Following this heady phase of rebirth is likely to be a quieter, introspective phase of Learning to Be Alone with Your New Self. Then the seeker moves on with greater insight to a Boldness to Dream. As the years add maturity, our need for meaning and relevance deepens. Those on the path to a more passionate life will likely move into a phase of Soul Seeking, where the emphasis is on gaining a deeper spiritual awareness. Ultimately, Seekers may graduate to Grandlove. The remainder of this book will explore each of these phases in greater detail with a variety of real-life stories as illustrations.

It is not unusual for a woman to plunge into the first romantic phase in her forties, perhaps precipitated by an unexpected divorce. Or it could begin for a woman with a newly emptied nest, when her husband takes her on a romantic holiday to celebrate her fiftieth birthday and she falls in love all over again.

We are just as susceptible to new romantic love in the middle of life as when we were in our twenties. The obsessive thinking is both exhilarating and humiliating: *Will he call? I don't care, oh, yes I do! This is ridiculous, I'm acting like a teenager, I'm a grown-up, I have grandchildren!* But we can't help it. The drive to love and be loved is so overwhelming; even with all the accumulated experience that one has by midlife, rational thought can hardly intervene when one is in the thrall of a Romantic Renaissance. The compulsive thoughts, the focused attention, the increased energy and loss of appetite and sleeplessness, the mood swings—from intense elation to gloom and doom—are disruptive to routine and responsible behavior.

They are the sweet sickness of romantic love.

The Drive to Love

Most of the Seekers I have interviewed desire reciprocal love even more than sex. Dr. Helen Fisher made headlines in *The New York Times* in 2005 with her study of how new love lights up the brain. She performed brain scans on college students in the throes of early-stage romantic love. She wanted to test a hunch.

"I thought this drive to love was one of the most powerful forces on earth," she says. "It's certainly more powerful than the sex drive. If you ask somebody to go to bed with you and they say, 'No thanks,' you don't kill yourself. But people in passionate love sometimes do kill themselves, or kill somebody else, or slip into a clinical depression, or stalk, when they have been rejected. The drive to love can be stronger than the will to live."

The same brain circuits are set off when you're 5 and you fall in love with a kid at your nursery school, or when you're 15 and you suddenly have a crush on a rock star, or when you're 85 and you fall in love again. The only difference among Dr. Fisher's younger respondents and those over 60 was that the older people did much more interesting things together. "They've got enough money to fly to Paris for the weekend, or go to the opera, or go tearing off down the Colorado River, whereas young people just don't have the resources."

The most important thing about early-stage intense romantic love is that it's a primitive motivational state. "It's about the motivation to win," as Dr. Fisher says. That intense goal orientation unleashes powerful emotions—euphoria, anxiety, obsessive thinking, paranoia—that stimulate even greater motivation to win the object of affection. Romantic love can be triggered at any age with just as much intensity as fear, joy, or sorrow. Dr. Fisher asserts that all those bored and desperate housewives whose marriages have become sexually moribund would light up if Prince Charming walked in the door.

I differ slightly. Prince Charming isn't going to just walk in the door. As I see it, a woman without a partner in middle life must be both hungry enough and bold enough to put effort into seeking a partner, or at least enough to put out signals that she is available.

Can a married woman and man enjoy a Romantic Renaissance in midlife? Of course. There are precious few long-term studies of how the central themes of midlife are negotiated by people in good marriages, but in my interviews with long-married couples they often describe a resurgence of romantic love and sexual intimacy once the children leave. As one husband said delightedly, "It's just about us again!"

This is one of the most striking and positive observations I found repeated again and again among happily seasoned couples, and it is backed up by solid evidence from psychologists I have interviewed. Once two people have been truly and passionately in love, that passion can be revived. Couples admit that they fall into and out of love and go through phases of boredom—it's part of the rhythm of life. But if ever chemistry has attracted a couple beyond all rational explanation, that romantic attraction can peak again.

Dr. Ethel Person, professor of clinical psychiatry at Columbia University and author of the classic book *Dreams of Love and Fateful Encounters: The Power of Romantic Passion,* is a convincing proponent of this thesis. "People can be angry at each other for a very long time, and then something will happen that they'll melt. It can be a threat, like an illness. Or it can be either a success or a setback, but something changes the equilibrium." It can be anything from a beautiful day when you happen to be together and it sparks a past memory that reactivates your feelings for each other. It can be around certain events that are shared joys, such as when something positive happens with a child. And it can be just any moment when you suddenly look at each other and understand something that's happening in the outside world—see eye to eye—in such a way that you remember the connections that brought you so close. It's all kinds of little things that can trigger those really early passionate feelings.

One long-married woman in her seventies told me, "Vacations do it for us. Having satisfying sex takes us so long at our age, that's the only place where we have enough time!"

A new lover, or a reignited romantic attraction, can be the impetus for a woman to seek out a new passion in life. Or it may give both partners the boldness to dream. "Knowing that you're really loved and appreciated, and feeling a deep love in return, is such a strengthening, reinforcing feeling, it gives you more courage about yourself in many ways," Dr. Person told me in an interview. Spouses who are secure in their own skin can be very supportive and proud of each other's achievements. A partner who believes in a woman's ability to master a new endeavor—without any concrete evidence that she can do it—and whose negative judgments can also be trusted as honest, is an enormous source of strength. That sense of endorsement gives many people the courage to push on with a new dream or endeavor.

Dr. Person argues eloquently for the transformative possibilities inherent in the experience of romantic love. "It is, in fact, an agent of change," she writes, creating "the impetus to begin new phases of life and undertake new endeavors. . . . In this way it resembles the great religious conversion experiences. Because of the identification with the person loved in a romantic relationship, we may even feel born again."

One of America's leading experts on marriage, psychologist Judith Wallerstein, asserts that "A richly rewarding and stable sex life is not just a fringe benefit. It is the central task of marriage." Dr. Wallerstein has been studying the same married and divorced couples in the Bay Area of California for thirty years. That rich, longitudinal view has convinced her that "sex serves a very serious function in maintaining both the quality and the stability of the relationship, replenishing emotional reserves and strengthening the marital bond." For her book *The Good Marriage,* she focused on fifty couples out of her study population in which each partner said separately that theirs was a great marriage. A revitalized sex life, she believes, is what refuels the marriages of those in or approaching midlife. But first, she warns, a couple has to renegotiate their relationship before they get to the sex. Finally, she makes her point with a sobering observation from her couples study:

> The greatest contrast between happily married and divorcing couples may well be in a domain of sex. By the time people file for divorce, sexual deprivation of several years' standing is shockingly common.

Costs and Benefits

Falling in romantic love with a new partner in midlife also comes with some costs. The body produces intense energy, you have a hard time sleeping, and you aren't much interested in eating. You can lose weight, which is nice, but you may feel alternately elated and exhausted. You don't go about your daily chores because you'd rather go out with your sweetheart; you'll make those business calls or phone the grandchildren later. Things remain undone.

Good stress comes out of romantic love as well. You're more likely to go to the gym. You have to go out and buy new clothes. You take better care of your grooming and maybe try a more fashionable hairstyle. You are more attractive to everybody, including yourself. You enjoy sex again. Good sex is good for you. Laughter is good for you. You take walks with your lover when you might have stayed home and curled up in front of the TV. The exercise is good for you. Novelty is especially good, and when you're falling in love, suddenly everything is novel. It renews your vitality.

Suddenly, you're happy in the grocery store and talk to the clerk, as opposed to being a grouch. Romantic love is a good stimulant for the brain, because you are being introduced to new things and new interests through your partner. You will probably read more. Your optimism can also spread into community activities and make you a more vital member of your society.

The most precious element of romantic love is making a real connection with a person who "gets you" and sees you in your best light. Suddenly, someone thinks you are the funniest thing, the smartest thing, the sexiest thing, the most charming thing. If your children are scandalized, let them know what a great boon this is to them. When you have a good companion, you're much nicer to be around. Your new self-sufficiency relieves much of the pressure on your adult children, who normally have to ask, "Is Mom all right?" "Do I have to spend the holidays with her again?" From a Darwinian perspective, your adult children should expend their energy on their own children—your grandchildren—not on you. Suddenly, at Christmastime, you won't be in their hair. You'll be off in Costa Rica with your sweetheart.

The first impetus to revitalize a deadened relationship, or escape from a dull state of singlehood, is likely to be lust. While religious conservatives define "lust" as sinful, I use the term here to mean the natural human desire for physical love. None of us is without it. Often, a seasoned woman's sexual longing is a dormant desire until awakened by some unexpected encounter. Maxine's story is a vivid illustration of how that pent-up desire can erupt when one least expects it.

Chapter 10

The Pilot Light Lover

*T*he tiny woman tucked into a sofa has an ethereal quality. Tendrils of platinum gray hair froth about her face and fall in wisps to her shoulders. Her face is powdery white and delicate as parchment but given focus by intense green eyes. Beneath her champagne-colored silk camisole, an ample bustline is lifted in an offertory angle.

Maxine drifted into her fifties leaving her sexual self behind, like reading glasses absentmindedly forgotten in another room. English-born, she had earlier enjoyed a respectably successful career as an opera singer in Vienna. Her love life was another story, plagued with mistakes and pitfalls. Her first love and marriage were to a man who was gay. They divorced after six years, and although they continue to have a loving and supporting friendship, he was hardly the partner for whom she longed. She did have a second husband, but, as she put it, "if you winked you missed him."

She worried about her marital failures. She worried even more about aging alone. "I didn't want to be sitting here in my fifties and a spinster," she confessed to a group that gathered with me at a home in the hills of Berkeley, California. "But I really only knew how to make love and dinner."

Upon moving from Vienna to the San Francisco Bay area some thirteen years before, Maxine had just about given up on finding the deep soul connection she was looking for. Her sex life dwindled to about the same frequency and quality as the singing opportunities she was being offered. And with the gradual loss of outlets for sexual pleasure in her two erogenous zones—her voice and her loins—she began to feel as cold as ashes.

The embers relit when Maxine was 52 and met the second love of her life on Match.com. For their second date he took her to a romantic dinner at a French restaurant where she found out he was the chef. He ordered her food. He held her hand under the table. She excused herself to go to the powder room.

"Just *thinking* about him, I felt myself lubricating like never before," she tells us, giggling and bringing forth murmurs of vicarious delight from the others. "I completely surrendered to this man. We were with each other practically twenty-four hours a day. I never thought, at fifty-two years of age, that it could happen. He was fifty-six, and *he* never thought it could happen. We fell almost instantly and deeply in love, and he certainly rose to the occasion!" She laughs wickedly. "In the third week of our romance, he whisked me off to the Ritz, in Paris. The city was melting under a heat wave, so we had to stay inside all the time, because the hotel had air-conditioning. It was probably the first time I'd had an orgasm."

The group found this revelation incredibly sad but not especially surprising; several of the other women admitted they hadn't known what they were missing in their former marriages until they felt a romantic rush in midlife.

At the time, Maxine was fending off the symptoms of menopause with a hormone gel. Her chef-lover had used Viagra. One night they stood on their hotel balcony and joined in a ceremonial tossing out of their sexual aids.

But Maxine's operatic story line took a sudden plot twist: "I lived in ecstasy for six months, and then he left me." She had become too voracious for his attentions.

Maxine admits being devastated. It took time for her to realize the gift he had left her.

Forget Devastate, Celebrate!

Maxine's chef is what I like to call the Pilot Light Lover, a transitional figure who appears in many of the stories of the Passionates I have interviewed. The Pilot Light Lover reignites a midlife woman's capacity for love and sex. Remember Carole, the full-figured divorcée whose first Internet lover assured her he liked big women? Like Maxine's chef, he gave Carole the confidence to invite a Romantic Renaissance, which led her to a candy jar full of interesting men who became lovers or friends.

Falling into romantic love after 50 makes a single woman feel very vulnerable, and for good reason. The Pilot Light Lover rarely lasts. He may be a married man disguised as single, or a great lover but unsuitable life partner—but so what? After the heartache wears off, a woman who is on her way to becoming seasoned should be able to celebrate the Pilot Light Lover's role in her journey. While the rush of a Romantic Renaissance can be as intense as romantic love was when we were young, we also possess half a lifetime of experience, and that gives us the ability to manage the delicious and dangerous turbulence. Just keep in mind that it is not wise to make any major life decisions when in this state of drunken bliss. The woman who does so may inhibit her transcendence into the next phase of the Passionate Life, stuck in the adolescent pattern of elation followed by despair and self-doubt.

The midlife woman must understand her power.

Maxine's eyes misted as she retold what she thought at the time was the end of the story. She put on her gold-framed reading glasses and read the first page of a proposed book that described how she had come out of the agony. The writing was powerful. She peeled off her glasses and faced us as candidly as she must have faced herself: "The answer was not in him. It is in me. 'Oh dear, I have to live inside myself.' " She was recognizing that she couldn't expect somebody else to complete her. She had to look into her dark corners and accept them. "I still feel fabulous as a woman." She brightened. "He didn't take that away from me. It's taken me fifty-three years to get to the place where I don't need a man's approval."

It's a cliché, but true: men can smell desperate from a mile away, especially men who may have fled an overly dependent wife or who are still tied to one through alimony payments. In a follow-up interview a year and a half after the romance with her Pilot Light Lover was extinguished, Maxine ruminated, "What I've learned is that when I'm in love, I'm just so intense . . . I got the message that I was too needy."

Maxine's renewed zest for life motivated her to find other outlets for her intensity. She sings in recitals and private homes, which provides a social network. She has also become a certified life coach and enjoys guiding people through the difficult transitions of their careers and love lives. Her new dream is to write a book reflecting on relationships. She still believes she will experience a mutually nurturing partnership. There's an apt analogy she uses to describe this calmer point in the romantic phase: "That love affair put sand into the oyster. I don't know that it's fully become a pearl yet, but it's starting to feel pearly!"

In the Romantic Renaissance phase, those of you who are initiators, Passionates, or Seekers—daring enough to step out into traffic, try a new pursuit, put yourself on the line, or put your profile online—will open up more possibilities, learn more about yourself, expand the range of your experience, and become more and more certain in following your instincts. You will also almost certainly make mistakes and maybe suffer heartbreaks, but we usually learn more from those than from our easy successes. If you see a man that in a blink you *know* you would connect with, would you go over and start the conversation? Or ask for his number getting off the plane after you have talked all through the flight? Would you consider a romance with a man ten years younger than you? Let's hear from some women who have tried it.

Chapter 11

Lusting After the Younger Lover

*J*anet Kiefer was too early a boomer to partake in the sexual revolution. She was a career military officer who married young and always played by the rules. When her husband left her for a younger woman, she was 48, and, as she now admits, "I became ill and thought I was going to die." She committed to excelling in her military career and eventually attained the rank of first lieutenant. Her confidence soared. So much so that one day, when she was 53, she was on the firing range qualifying with her weapon when she noticed a handsome young officer next to her. She introduced herself, and they chatted while reloading. He was on the quiet side. So when they went off the firing line to wait for the next round, she walked over to him and touched his arm.

"I'm sorry if I invaded your space," she said. He laughed and said it wasn't a problem. Several weeks passed before she happened to be at the academy for inspection and suddenly the young officer appeared. Again they exchanged a few words. A couple of days later her phone rang. It was the young officer asking her out.

She knew the age gap was large—it turned out to be twenty years—so she said no, but her body felt weightless and her heart was racing with *yes, yes*. A couple of days passed, and her phone rang again. And again. He called three times asking her to change her mind. She did. When they met at a poolside restaurant, he had a table with two beers waiting and a bouquet of roses. She was astonished to feel totally relaxed with him, and he seemed to feel the same way. "It was as though we had known each other forever and met in another life." When they kissed good night, they both knew instantly what was going to happen.

"I experienced sex that night in ways that I did not know were possible," says the lieutenant. "I became completely free with this young man and allowed him to pleasure me and to show me how to pleasure him. That was five years ago. He basically has shown me how to be sexually free and to try new and different things without any embarrassment or shame. Now, at the age of fifty-eight, I don't kid myself. I do realize that someday my wrinkles will become deeper, my breasts will drop, my stomach might get pouchy, and the younger man will look elsewhere. But right now I am enjoying this fantastic sexual time in my life where I am finding climax can happen more than once a night or day."

A Worldwide Trend

Weird? No, not even unusual. Around the world, more and more seasoned women are feeling free to date younger men. As many as a third of unmarried American women who are dating in their forties through their sixties are going out with younger men, according to *AARP Magazine*'s 2003 survey. And why not? More than two thirds of men in this age group said they were dating younger women. There is enough of a subculture now of older women hooking up with much younger men to spawn a website: AgelessLove.com.

These women are by and large not widows, they are mostly divorced boomers who have already raised their children and are more emotionally and economically independent than young women. They are risk takers like Carlene, the latter-day Amelia Earhart who lives with her much younger flyboy lover. But they also include more conventional women like Lieutenant Kiefer. A lusty interlude with a young lover can peel away rigid inhibitions.

Many single women have had their fill of high-maintenance husband care and voice a ubiquitous complaint about their first marriage: *no emotional intimacy.* They are looking for fun, flirtation, somebody to notice and appreciate or even idealize them; somebody who shares *their* interests or maybe turns them on to new ones; somebody who isn't threatened by *their* accomplishments or dreams. And many are unabashedly hungry for good sex. After all, these women belong to the pioneer generation that brought us the sexual revolution, although many missed out on its permission to experiment. Why give up now? Those who seize the opportunity tell me they often realize, in retrospect, how valuable it was to have a "transitional affair" with a younger lover who appreciates an older woman for her worldliness and reminds her that her erotic self still lives!

They have also been liberated by the ease of meeting men online. They never would have felt comfortable sitting in bars or cruising church socials to find male company. But being able to test out a dozen different men in one night through online conversations, before even choosing to meet one for coffee, eliminates the tedium of a two-hour dinner with a dork.

In a book published in 2000, *Older Women, Younger Men,* the young male interviewees spell out what attracts them: "The ability to talk about anything." "Never boring." "[She] offered me space, devotion, and herself, which I couldn't find in anyone else. She reflects back to me what a good person I am, which builds my confidence and self-esteem." "Just the fact there's so much to learn from an older woman, that they have so many more life experiences to draw upon . . . it's like a rush." "She helped me to grow up." "Emotional stability." "Calm." According to the authors, Susan Winter and Felicia Brings, all the men to whom they talked commented that sex with older women was better. "She knows what she wants and how to communicate that to a partner." And the man is rewarded by knowing he is appreciated as a good lover.

Another plus is not having to worry about an unwanted pregnancy. Dennis Watlington, a playwright and filmmaker who was quite a sexual athlete in his salad days, has a very different outlook now that he has reached 50. "Don't even show up unless you have your postmenopausal papers stamped. That means your children are grown or they're heading out the door—wonderful! I just want you, and what we have to share."

Interestingly, marriage to a much younger man seems to have an impact on a woman's longevity. Researchers at the University of Oklahoma, using data from the U.S. Census and U.S. Center for Health Statistics, studied women between the ages of 50 and 75 whose husbands were between six to fourteen years younger. Thirty percent of those wives lived longer than expected.

Hollywood Catches On

It took moviemakers a while to catch up to this worldwide trend and overcome Hollywood's congenital resistance to casting seasoned female stars in romantic roles. *Something's Gotta Give* was the breakthrough. Diane Keaton, playing a postmenopausal playwright, does nothing overtly seductive. She's 50-something, thin, rich, and famous, and describes herself as "strong, controlling, know-it-all, neurotic, but kind of cute." Jack Nicholson, playing the paunchy playboy who lusts after her 20-year-old daughter, played by Amanda Peet, is titillated by Diane's teasing. Keanu Reeves, as the drop-dead handsome young doctor, ignores the daughter and pursues Keaton like a lovesick puppy.

Can you believe this?

What is the allure of the older single woman, personified by Keaton (who is, in real life, 58 years old)? Beneath the age lines clearly etched in her face and the turtlenecks pulled up to her chin, what does her character have that her adorable, dewy-skinned daughter does not?

She's a head trip. Funny, sharp-tongued, she is self-mocking, even as she is able to poke fun at the ego bubble around a man's head. "I'm not regular," she tells Nicholson. "And men want regular." Ah, but that is the fascination of the seasoned woman. She has been uniquely shaped by her life experiences, and, like a flowering shrub pruned over many seasons, she stands out.

She doesn't *need* a man, or at least not for the things many young women are looking for: money, status, babies, security. Men in their thirties or forties find it a relief to be with a woman whose personality is formed, who knows who she is, and stands in contrast to the nervous push-pull of a younger woman who isn't secure yet in her own identity or who, when the alarm on her biological clock goes off, pursues him with the zeal of a sperm hunter.

When I spoke at a conference of 450 women over the age of 45 in Orange County, California, all members of the Web network WomanSage, I asked the audience how many had seen *Something's Gotta Give*. Almost every hand went up, and ripples of pleasure spread through the room. "How many of you would have chosen the young doctor played by Keanu over the Jack Nicholson character who was her age?" A forest of hands shot up for Keanu.

"And how many of you would have chosen Jack?" Only three hands went up.

Aspects of the Keaton character are based on the real-life experience of the screenwriter and director, Nancy Meyers. When I interviewed Meyers, she revealed what she has learned about the attraction of older women for younger men like the character played by Keanu. "He's the anti-Jack. He's generationally so different. He's a younger guy who had a younger mother and was not brought up the way Jack was. He doesn't have those hang-ups." In real life, Meyers says, "Keanu really looks up to and admires Diane Keaton, she's an icon. While Jack looks upon her as a pal."

Young men have always been fascinated by accomplished older women, whose high status gilds them with an aura of glamour. The young Keanu character is infatuated with the playwright played by Keaton because of her fame and the world she lives in, as well as her beauty and sexiness. The younger man doesn't have to feel competitive with such a woman. He is still in the apprentice stage of building his career. He isn't expected to be able to pick up the check in swanky restaurants.

"He's interested in her mind," says Meyers. "He keeps saying she's brilliant. Her accomplishments are not threatening to him—that was a point I wanted to make—because after all this time, after all the literature and talking and therapy, our accomplishments still *are* threatening to our own generation of men."

Moving Beyond the Vanity Crisis

Feeling lustful attraction to younger men is only one phase of the Romantic Renaissance. It may lead to a transformative romance, or it may just play itself out in fantasy and a few flirtations. If it helps in overcoming the inevitable vanity crisis that seizes almost all women—and men—it has served a purpose. As men have long known, it's a salve to the narcissistic wound of getting older and feeling invisible or taken for granted.

It must be said that it's tough to have sexual confidence over 50.

When the magic moment does come, most older women can't think of anything but the embarrassment of exposing their expanded girth and sagging treasures. But an affair often spurs a woman on to make serious changes in her weight and appearance, which are appreciated and affirmed by her younger lover, and the whole cycle is reinforced: she *is* younger than she looks, in face and body as well as spirit.

The real "click" for a woman may happen *after* the transitional affair, when she meets an accomplished man close to her own age. It's a relief to talk to somebody who shares the same cultural history, who remembers being thrilled by the Beatles, and who is comfortable enough to trade reading glasses in a restaurant. A boy-man may worship your self-possession and success in life, but he must seek those things for himself—he cannot absorb them from you by osmosis.

Marrying the Younger Lover

Terry McMillan knows the pitfalls of succumbing to the apparent worship of a boy-man. She was already a millionaire and the celebrated author of a best-selling novel made into the movie *Waiting to Exhale,* when she was beguiled by a 20-year-old Jamaican boy she met at a resort on the island. She was 42 at the time. He made her believe he was crazy about her, she says. She married him in Maui three years later, and they settled in her $4 million home outside San Francisco. The author celebrated their match in her next novel, *How Stella Got Her Groove Back,* the thinly fictionalized story of a single African-American mother's torrid romance with a Jamaican young enough to be her son.

The fairy-tale romance ended six years later. In June 2005, Terry McMillan very publicly accused her husband of having based their marriage on a "fraud," marrying her only to gain U.S. citizenship and never telling her until she confronted him that he was gay. "It was devastating to discover that a relationship I had publicized to the world as life-affirming and built on mutual love was actually based on deceit," she wrote in her filing for divorce. "I was humiliated." The famous author was ordered to pay her husband $2,000 a month in spousal support plus $25,000 in attorneys' fees until a full trial is held to determine the validity of a restrictive prenuptial agreement.

Other celebrities partnered with younger men seem to have more enduring relationships, from Demi Moore to Julianne Moore and Madonna to Candace Bushnell, the creator of *Sex and the City,* who told Oprah Winfrey that "one of the reasons why my marriage works is that it's not a traditional kind of marriage. My husband is ten years younger."

＊　　＊　　＊

There always exists, of course, the possibility of true love. And like all good relationships, what often helps transcend the initial infatuation is a shared interest; Melodee Touma is a good example. She is the mother of four sons and was in the midst of a separation from her husband of seventeen years when she entered a Yahoo! chat room for French speakers. She had lived in France briefly in her twenties and was hoping to brush up on her skills.

There she began chatting with a 21-year-old Frenchman named Jeremy. He was engaged, and Melodee had no romantic interest in this young man, but they enjoyed talking. They liked the same music. They would send each other copies of their favorite songs. He practiced his English and she her French. She was able to reminisce with him about her days in France. And despite Jeremy's age, Melodee found him to be a mature conversationalist. "He listened to me when I talked, and he responded. It's something I find to be really rare in men I've met."

After four months of conversational friendship, both Jeremy and Melodee were feeling sparks, though neither said anything of their feelings. When Jeremy came to the United States to visit family and study English, he arranged to visit Melodee in Petaluma, California.

She was nervous while driving to the airport. Of course they were just friends, she told herself, and he was so young. But she had taken an unusually long time to dress that morning. She wore her long blond hair down and loose and was dressed casually, but attractively, in jeans.

The first time they saw each other was a shock. After four months of speaking, they'd come to have mental images of each other. The Jeremy who came off the plane had very short hair and very thick glasses. "He looked a little nerdy."

She approached Jeremy and gave him an awkward hug. His mouth was open. "Oh," he said. "I had no idea you were so . . ."

There was a pause. "Do you mean to say 'fat'?" Melodee asked him. *"Non. Maigre,"* he said shyly in French. Meaning skinny.

Melodee was surprised, but pleasantly. She was only a size four, but her mind-set had been shaped by having been married to a man who preferred her to be a size two.

Things became romantic, despite her initial impression that he wasn't her type. The sex was fantastic, which surprised Melodee. "When I was married, I honestly thought I had become frigid. I'd lost all interest in sex. I had all these hormone tests. I think it was just that my ex-husband was mean; it shut me down, physically and emotionally." Jeremy, on the other hand, offered Melodee an emotional intimacy she had lacked in her marriage. In no time, they were in love.

Many of Melodee's friends raised their eyebrows when she told them she was getting married again, and to whom. Her own mother was dismissive: "He's just looking for another momma." But four years into their marriage, the couple is still together and Melodee's mother has changed her opinion. "He's the mature, stable one!" her mother claims. Melodee agrees. "I'm much more spontaneous and impulsive. But he's teaching me, and I'm twenty-six years older than him!"

The economic differential that often sets such a couple apart is not an issue with this pair. Jeremy works in retail, and Melodee has some stocks and savings. Their income isn't much, especially in contrast with that of Melodee's first husband, who earned more than $200,000 a year, but they are content with it. "We both just want a simple life," says Melodee. "Neither of us is attracted by the idea of a high-powered job."

Of course there are some aspects of this unusual partnership that are challenges to both of them. Melodee worries that as she gets older Jeremy may want to leave her for someone with fewer wrinkles and more years left. He insists he doesn't notice the wrinkles. "And I couldn't be attracted to anyone else," he tells her. "They're not you." Jeremy thinks that one day he might like to expand their family. "My husband would be so happy to have a child with me," Melodee recognizes. "But I've had my family." They're discussing international adoption.

These are concerns that can surface in even the most traditional of couples. Melodee and Jeremy both believe they are manageable, especially given the solid foundation on which their marriage is based. Neither had an obvious neurotic need for an other to fill some void in themselves. They became friends first through a shared love of a language and a culture. They were able to get over those superficial first physical impressions because there was a common interest.

Chapter 12

Menopausal Sex—Grin or Bear It?

"*I* started having hot flashes in my late forties, so I started cooking with tofu and drinking soy shakes and getting really healthy, but I wasn't expecting the changes in my sexual response," said the petite hypnotherapist, commanding the immediate attention of the Berkeley group of midlife daters. With two marriages long behind her, she had not had sex for a number of years.

"Then my younger Latin lover came back into my life after that long, dry period without sex," she said. "I was so tight, it hurt! But I just pretended I was a virgin again."

Hilarity broke out. It was fun to hear a woman put a grin on the common dread of bearing up under painful postmenopausal sex. But it's not a laughing matter when making love becomes so painful, the partners can't pretend anymore. Leslie Ann admitted that her "revirgination" did not prolong their brief obsession. She asked him to go.

Consider that an estimated 50 million American women are somewhere in the menopausal transition or postmenopausal. This should be a significant enough population to demand clear and accurate information. But roughly every ten years our scientific and medical establishments reverse their "findings." This chapter will try to clarify some of the confusion, particularly as it impacts on the quality of a woman's sexual life.

Most American women transit the menopausal passage somewhere between the ages of 40 and 58, with a median age of 52. Menopause can be the bridge to the most vital and liberated period in a woman's life, but the bridge usually does cross turbulent waters. Hormones have a powerful effect on our physical life and our mood. The great majority of women experience hot flashes, night sweats, vaginal dryness, and sleep disturbances. In addition, mood swings are estimated by different studies to affect up to one-fifth of women in the perimenopausal phase (the period leading up to menopause when the menstrual cycle is erratic) and up to two thirds of women in postmenopause. Most of these effects are temporary. But two of them become increasingly common, and troubling, throughout the menopausal transition: sleep interruptions and vaginal dryness.

"Honey, I Love You a Lot, but Can We Save It?"

This was a prime concern of a group of academic women who met with me in a university town in a medium-sized midwestern city. Toni was the most striking woman in the room: tall, with a statuesque body and girlish sweep of honey brown hair, she is the wife of the university provost. All the other women admired her and her marriage, and it was easy to see why: she is naturally gregarious and radiates life. Since the university is the only public institution in town, her husband has a visible role in advocating for the university and Toni enjoys playing her part as a hostess. Her younger assistant gushes, "You guys have such a great marriage, you're a great team."

Although Toni is only six years younger than her second husband, they are reflections of different cultural eras. His children always say, "Hey Dad, how come Toni gets our music and you don't?" The biggest difference is in their sexual experience. Toni and her first husband had declared an open marriage—very *au courant* in that last round of the Sixties bacchanalia before the AIDS epidemic—but like most such experiments, their open marriage ended in a jealous divorce. As a committed feminist, Toni worked with a sense of ideological mission at locating the orgasmic response and learning how to reproduce it with or without a partner. When she met her second husband, she was the returning graduate student and he was the older professor. Being a rather starchy academic type, he was intrigued by her sexual forthrightness. Once they had both overcome their fears of repeating divorce, they married. By now she is 56 and he is 61.

"Now that we've been together for twenty-two years," she tells the group, "the whole sex thing for us is finding time when we're both not too tired or too committed to other things. Orgasm is not the main thing now. What I really enjoy about a sexual relationship is the feeling of closeness."

A doubtful divorcée poses a troubling question: "But is that enough for a man?"

"Well, it's more, um, more physically difficult for both of us than it was twenty years ago," Toni demurs. She adds hastily, "It's still very important and rewarding as an expression of our intimacy and commitment. We share more talk now than lovemaking. We talk about my father's failing health or whether to put down our old dog."

Another woman presses the point: "Is that enough for *you*?"

I glance down at her questionnaire. In response to the question "How do you feel about sex after 50?" she checked, "Never give up."

In a subsequent private interview, guaranteed anonymity, Toni admits the challenge she is facing in postmenopause: "There's one thing in our relationship that bothers me—when I say no to sexual relations. Now, in our later stages of life, Hugh is much more eager for sexual activity than I am—the roles are reversed. For him, I think, it's a way of reestablishing our connection. He probably also needs assurance that he's still active and desired. My problem is, I've experienced strong physical changes with menopause—hot flashes, a significant decline in my libido, and some pain with intercourse, because of dryness. All the lubricants in the world don't seem to help. And my doctor won't give me hormones because I have fibroid cysts in my uterus."

Another dampener on her desire is the deterioration in her own self-image since menopause. "I do find I look less attractive to myself than I did," she acknowledges. "I ran a lot of miles in my thirties and forties and now I have some early osteoporosis, so I'll probably have to throw out the pointy girl shoes I love so much. I look at myself in the mirror and see parts of my face are drooping. My coloring is fading, so I have to be more careful about not looking overly made up. I'm heavier. Hugh claims he finds me sexier than ever. The irony is, I don't *feel* as sexy because I don't feel as attractive.

"One of the things I find myself saying is, 'Honey, I love you a lot, but can we save it?' He laughs and says yes. Sometimes I manage to participate even though I'd rather not." At the end of our interview, Toni discloses what she cannot tell her husband. "Here's the truth, and he would be very hurt to know it: I could probably go for a year without making love to my husband and not miss it."

We're Older Now, What Do You Expect?

There may be no more toxic a myth to middle- and later-life love than the notion that sex is over after 50, or that a husband or wife will be willing to "save it" indefinitely. Romantic love has a regrettably short shelf life. For a long-lasting monogamous marriage to tolerate the inevitable stresses and temptations of life, it needs to be enlivened by flashes of passion, fantasy, fun, mystery, and a dependable intimacy. By dependable, I don't mean the kind of perfunctory sex dispensed a couple of times a month, on demand, to keep the old boy calmed down but devoid of passion or much emotional content. I mean conscious, creative efforts to find the time and desire for "love moments."

Sex certainly isn't the only thing that holds a marriage together, but its absence can loosen the bond. When sexual closeness is offered with the kind of forethought and delight in preparation one would bring to fixing a sumptuous meal for a new lover, it may not have to be shared often to be memorable. The memory of great love moments can be endlessly replayed by both partners, during separations and the inevitable periods of abatement of desire or illness. We don't easily forget those occasions when sexual union releases us from the cage of self and allows us to feel a merging of souls.

Woe, then, to the woman or man who dismisses sex by mouthing the old rationale: *We're older now, what do you expect?* Several sex counselors I interviewed, who deal primarily with working-class women, relate a common attitude among women over 50: when their husbands ask for sex, they see it as just one more annoying demand. Many carry layers of resentment for having pulled so much of the load in their marriages. They've never had particularly satisfying sex lives, they're tired, and if they didn't have a high sex drive earlier in life, they may not have much left at all in middle life. Their husbands become sexual beggars. The wives find plenty of cultural support for the view that their husbands are being piggish: *Why doesn't he understand we don't have to do it anymore after 50?* Often, say the sex counselors, these women have no concept that there might be some physical change in their bodies that diminishes their sexual appetite or comfort. They just don't make the connection with the menopausal transition and so do nothing to ameliorate the changes.

Let's consider the other extreme: women who have always enjoyed sex and who are surprised and dismayed by the changes that occur during the menopausal transition. They may have a new lover or a new marriage or be dating, and they want to be just as easily aroused and satisfied as when they were in their twenties, without acknowledging that nothing in the body stays the same.

My generation was herded en masse onto hormone replacement therapy (HRT). By the year 2000, 6 million menopausal women were using HRT to relieve hot flashes and night sweats, sleep and mood disturbances, and vaginal dryness. We loved the promise that those little pills would keep us young indefinitely, and we felt justified by assurances from our doctors that using HRT would protect us against the number one female killer, heart disease, as well as the dreaded bone crusher, osteoporosis. We also knew, from comparing the appearance of older friends, that those using HRT often have smoother skin, glossier hair, fuller lips, and an indefinable light behind the eyes that is a tip-off to continued sexual vitality.

In 2002, a bombshell exploded in the face of this conventional wisdom when the Women's Health Initiative (WHI) suddenly suspended its trial of the standard hormone replacement therapy (Prempro, a combination of estrogens and progestin). It was found that this preparation not only did not prevent heart disease, but in a small number of women it can exacerbate underlying cardiovascular risk factors and lead to stroke or heart attack.

These alarming results have only recently been placed in better perspective. If you thought this study proved that hormones are bad for most menopausal women, you can think it through again. The average profile among the sixteen thousand subjects was a 60-year-old woman, most of whom had no symptoms. They were started on hormone therapy well after menopause *for the first time,* to find out if it would decrease their risk of heart attack and stroke and what impact it had on their risk of breast and colon cancer. What relevance did this study have for those boomer women who are only now crossing the bridge into the menopausal passage—women who are now between their mid-forties and mid-fifties? This is the most symptomatic group, and also the age group whose absolute risk for heart attacks and breast cancer is low. They were minimally represented in the study.

Dr. Wulf Utian, executive director of the North American Menopause Society (NAMS) and professor emeritus at Case Western Reserve University, points out that most women in the 50-to-60 study group in the WHI trial actually showed a *decrease* in heart disease while on HRT. That part of the study was never publicized. And the more subtle issues of quality of life in the menopausal years—mood, memory, energy, and sexual satisfaction—were given short shrift. Dr. Utian is also critical of the memory portion of the study, which concluded that hormone therapy did not protect against age-related changes in the brain. "The explanation for the negative WHI results is that most of the women studied were started on hormone replacement therapy beyond the age of sixty-five, much too far after menopause."

But most people read only the headlines. And the scary headlines created panic and overreaction. The more militant antihormone proponents among the researchers defended themselves by asserting that HRT, when compared to a placebo, provided "no improvement in emotional stability, cognitive function, sleep, or sexual satisfaction."

This is false.

Many women loudly protested. "Three weeks after I went off HRT, I felt depressed and foggy" was a common complaint. There are clearly many women who notice a change in sleep, mood, cognitive functioning, and vaginal dryness, all related to their postmenopausal lowered estrogen levels.

Helen Fisher, the anthropologist we heard from earlier in connection with her study on how new love lights up the brain, puts her finger on a key point that was absent in the report and headlines: "The Women's Health Initiative never said the important thing, which is that estrogen helps with orgasm." Dr. Fisher speaks as a researcher as well as from personal experience. Five years ago she fell in love with a new man. Sex was wonderful, and orgasms were easily achieved. She put herself through the brain-scanning machine that she was using to measure the cortical activity of college-aged women and men in romantic love to see how her own midlife passion stacked up against theirs. "Mine was off the charts!" she found. Sex was so good with her new love, she decided to experiment with cutting her low-dose estrogen budget in half. (She was using the Vivelle 0.05 milligram transdermal patch.)

Instead of changing her patch twice a week, she changed it only once. Everything else stayed constant—she remained just as in love, her lover was just as ardent, no unusual stresses in life. But within three or four weeks, Helen was dismayed to notice that she couldn't reach orgasm—with her new lover or on her own. That's when she concluded, "It's the estrogen that governs the actual sexual response."

I asked Dr. Utian, director of NAMS, to comment on that conclusion. "There is evidence suggesting that estrogen enhances sexuality in women," he says. "If you think about women's sexual response during the reproductive cycle, estrogen reaches a peak at day fourteen of the twenty-eight-day cycle, at point of ovulation. That's when female animals are most receptive to intercourse and will actually court the males. But as the estrogen level goes down and progesterone kicks in, the whole response turns off again."

Dr. Pat Allen, guru gynecologist to thousands of New York's menopausal women, states from her clinical experience, "Vaginal estrogen is absolutely necessary for comfortable sex after menopause in almost all women. It's necessary for the vagina to be supple, vascularized, moist." But she cautions that Helen's story does not mean that menopausal women need to use *systemic* hormone therapy in order to be orgasmic and have a continuing sexual life. "When the effect of diminished estrogen becomes apparent to a woman in the menopausal transition—if she experiences more difficulty achieving orgasm or discomfort during intercourse—the treatment is very simple and seems to be safe. She can apply a lima-bean-sized amount of estradiol cream directly to the clitoris." (Estrace is the name of the commercial product.)

In addition, many gynecologists, including Dr. Allen, favor the increasingly well accepted medication Vagifem. It is a tiny estrogen tablet that has been specially formulated to be inserted into the vagina. It acts locally on the genital tissue, but little is absorbed into the bloodstream, so it does not carry the risks presented by systemic hormone therapy. Within the first few weeks of application, the tissues of the vagina should be nicely estrogenized and intercourse becomes more comfortable, provided the woman has not gone too long without hormones or activity.

"I see little reason not to use vaginal estrogen two or three times a week, low dose," agrees Dr. Utian. "In my opinion, the risk factors are pretty close to zero." The use of a vibrator can also become an important aid to enhancing a woman's capacity to achieve orgasm. The more she practices on her own and teaches her partner, the easier it is for her to reach climax. Elegant new variations on this old-fashioned device have become so well accepted that they are now sold in upscale boutiques such as Myla on Madison Avenue, and written up in *The New York Times.*

Dr. Utian is very uncomfortable with the new conventional wisdom that women who've gone off hormones and are having terrible menopausal symptoms should be given antidepressants. "It takes us back to prehormone days when women were told, 'Your menopausal maladies are all in your mind,' " he says. "We don't have any lengthy enough studies on the effect of giving antidepressants to women who aren't depressed. We know that when a patient stops taking an antidepressant, there is a withdrawal effect, so it changes brain chemistry. Are we right to change the brain chemistry of a woman who isn't depressed? Or make her dependent on an antidepressant?"

So much of sex for the seasoned woman depends upon her willingness to address her health issues head-on. There is no reason why a woman like Toni, the university provost's wife who loves her husband and who enjoyed sex until after menopause, should tell him to "save it" and deny both of them the delight of physical affection. In fact, after being urged to find a different doctor, Toni began seeing a female internist who recommended a low-dose vaginal cream. "I have noticed a change in my libido and in my comfort during intercourse," Toni wrote to tell me. "This doctor is great to talk to, and my desire level has improved—it's a world of difference."

Fight It or Flow with It?

Now back to the menopause basics. The rough part of the transition may be only a matter of months. When and if a woman is in it, she'll know. Now is the time to make an alliance with her body for the future. She will need to sleep more, because her usual night's sleep may be interrupted by sweats. It helps to eat earlier, which makes her metabolism more efficient. My advice is, don't fight it.

Take the pause.

Even if it means temporarily cutting back on working at your usual pace, it is important to listen to the cues from your body, just as it was when you were pregnant. Better to leave work a little early and take a nap before dinner than to go to a business cocktail party and break out in hot flashes that send you to the bar, screaming, "Where's the ice water?" You may find yourself weepy for no particular reason. Or rather, for a reason so deep in your unconscious, you may not connect it with your mood. You are grieving. This is a loss, an emptying of your magical capacity to give life. But that emptying also frees up enormous energy and allows a more singular focus on things you have always wanted to do.

Because menopause is as individual as a thumbprint, it requires a lot of reading and experimentation to become conversant with your midlife mental, physical, and sexual circuitry. Women determined to continue pursuing a passionate life listen to their bodies and try to be vigilant about monitoring their health—making use of natural botanical agents and nutritional supplements, alternating between weight-bearing exercise to keep their bones strong, yoga practice, and Pilates to build core strength and retain flexibility, and practicing meditation to cultivate serenity. The greatest benefit of such efforts is "postmenopausal zest." That term, coined by the pioneering anthropologist Margaret Mead, has been affirmed by millions of women who continue to be amazed upon entering a new stage of equilibrium. Moving from perimenopause into menopause—the cessation of menstrual periods—and later settling into the calm of postmenopause is usually a full seven-year transition, like most other major life passages. The reward is release to pursue the passion of your Second Adulthood.

All Choices Have Consequences

Many women I meet around the country have confided the same secret: they have chosen to restart systemic hormone therapy. Or, as one attractive TV personality in her early sixties put it, "I graze now and then, just to keep myself sexually toned." Doctors also tell me they have been bombarded by requests from women to "go back on," but they encourage patients to use a much lower dose and under a much more watchful eye than before.

To counter the firestorm of protests over the peremptory results of the WHI trial, the National Institutes of Health appointed an independent panel of experts to produce a more definitive statement of what works and what is safe. The NIH report, released in March 2005, acknowledged what most women have known all along: nothing is as effective as estrogen therapy for alleviating menopausal symptoms—and 25 percent of women continue to have moderate to severe symptoms into postmenopause. More pertinent, the panel recognized that smaller doses of hormone therapy (roughly one quarter the strength of Prempro) actually have a good effect on older women. The Nurses' Health Study, which has tracked the health of 121,701 registered nurses since 1976, reports that women who remained on low doses versus women who took the higher standard doses had fewer heart attacks, fewer strokes, and less risk of blot clots.

"Low-dose estrogen" was quantified by the panel to mean less than, or equal to, 0.3 milligrams of Premarin (which produces a spike of hormone in the bloodstream and is metabolized by the liver over the course of only a few hours); or 0.5 milligrams of oral micronized estradiol; or 0.025 milligrams a day of transdermal estradiol (as in the lowest dose of the Vivelle-Dot or Climara patch). The old standard dose of Premarin— 0.625 milligrams—has been found to increase the risk of developing serious disease.

A woman needs to evaluate her own relative risks for long-term negative health effects against the benefits of short-term use of low-dose hormone replacement for symptom management. If she is well into her fifties and has a family history of heart attacks at early ages, blood clots, or strokes, or her mother or other close relatives had premenopausal breast cancer, her risks in using systemic hormone therapy must be seriously evaluated. On the other hand, if a woman is 48 with no history of heart disease or breast cancer in her family, and she is eating sensibly, exercising, and not obese, but she finds perimenopause is causing misery—emotional ups and downs, memory lapses, foggy thinking, and/or lost libido—Dr. Utian and Dr. Allen agree that a few years of hormone therapy will probably enhance her quality of life with very little health risk.

Beware the New Snake Oil Salespeople

The investigators at the WHI dumped their results on the public without giving medical professionals time to review the results and reorient their patients. As a result, the study has triggered a lot of anger and distrust by women of their traditional doctors. And doctors are reluctant to prescribe hormones "off label" because of increasingly rigid warnings from their malpractice insurers. So what's happening?

A cottage industry of "alternative medicine" practitioners and spa-like clinics has sprung up to cater to women who are clamoring for "natural" and "off-label" preparations. These women will often pay a hefty fee out of pocket for a consultation or even "self-refer" to a practitioner who will take the time to listen to their complaints over the phone: "I have hot flashes, I can't sleep through the night, and my libido is shot."

The patient is usually told she can order a saliva test to measure her hormone levels. Then the practitioner will prescribe the "bioidentical" hormone cocktail she needs and have it compounded for her by a special pharmacy. Women are given the impression that the cream or gel or lotion or capsule is the equivalent of what the body would make and at a level that will bring them back to "normal." Therefore, it must be safe. And unlike what traditional gynecologists are giving them, they are told these "bioidentical" hormones won't cause breast cancer, heart attacks, or strokes.

The fallacy is that a woman of reproductive years who is producing a normal balance of estrogen, progesterone, and testosterone has "levels" that fluctuate moment to moment, day to day, week to week. There is never a standard level in the body. Saliva tests are useless, according to scientific experts. The term "bioidentical" is a great marketing phrase, but in medical terms, it is virtually meaningless.

The nontraditional health practitioners who are selling women estrogen and testosterone in privately mixed creams and gels and pellets are playing into their magical thinking. "If it's not a pill, it's not a drug— that's the lie too many women buy," says Dr. Allen. "But these *are* drugs, and they *do* have consequences."

Estradiol is the only form of estrogen that matches what the body produces. It is available in doses that are approved by the FDA to provide a satisfactory blood level. And it is available in all the same forms in commercially produced products—in the Vivelle patch and in the lotion form, Estrasorb, and the gel form, Estragel. Dr. Utian says that these products have been through the safety and efficacy studies that the FDA requires for approval. "The mixtures created at the compounding pharmacies have never gone through the FDA process, and there are no inspectors stopping by to randomly test for batch-to-batch differences, as they do with the pharmaceutical manufacturers."

A Topper of Testosterone?

Testosterone is the hormone of desire for both women and men. Procter & Gamble's study of a testosterone patch established that the drug increases women's sexual desire and satisfaction. Women who wore a dummy testosterone patch also showed a strong response to the placebo, which may be due to the increased learning curve about their own bodies that participants in such a study often enjoy. Doctors who participated in the trial, such as Dr. Lila E. Nachtigall, a veteran gynecologist and reproductive endocrinologist at the New York University School of Medicine, were favorably impressed with the patch. With more than twenty years of experience in prescribing various hormone therapies to her patients, Dr. Nachtigall was hoping finally to have a solution to offer to countless patients who complain of loss of libido.

"We're the only mammal that outlives its reproductive functions," she says. She points out that nature made us to live only about fifty years, but since technology has stretched out our life cycle, we must rethink our priorities. "Are we entitled to have everything at eighty that we had at forty? Well, I don't know, but I could see wanting it."

The FDA turned down P&G's first application for approval of its eagerly anticipated patch. Ever since, women have been taking matters into their own hands. Some nurse practitioners I have interviewed are willing to offer out-of-state patients advice over the phone. Women can get prescriptions for "off-label" testosterone as a cream, lotion, gel, injections, or subcutaneous pellets, despite the fact that there are absolutely no long-term data on the safety or efficacy of testosterone in women. Prescriptions for testosterone in these various non-pill forms rose eightfold between 1999 and 2004.

"It blows my mind that savvy women who used to come in to the traditional physician's office with all sorts of intelligent questions about the risks and benefits of hormones," says Dr. Utian, "are willing to subject themselves to some experimental mixture of estrogen or testosterone prescribed by someone over the phone. What are these women thinking? By the time they're showing mustaches and getting deep voices, they've probably already done some damage to their cardiovascular system."

Many women are quite sensible about using a small amount of testosterone as a topper. But more and more women are borrowing their husbands' testosterone patches and cutting them in half.

"Self-medicating with your husband's testosterone patch is dangerous and foolish," warns Dr. Laurie Romanzi, another New York gynecologist who participated in P&G's trials on the testosterone patch for women. "Male-dose patches will severely overdose any woman who uses them," she warns. "Testosterone overdose may cause not only mustaches but permanent deepening of the voice, permanent abnormal enlargement of the clitoris, flattening of the breasts, acne, weight gain, and raging mood swings."

Dr. Utian draws an analogy to all of the athletes taking androgenic steroids. When a man is given more testosterone than he needs, his muscles bulge up and he'll probably break some records, but he risks sudden death syndrome during training from the damage done to his cardiovascular system. "Women who are taking way more testosterone than they should are making themselves guinea pigs. And we don't even know if lowered testosterone is responsible for their lack of libido."

P&G is continuing to do safety trials on its patch, which is under simultaneous consideration for approval by American, Canadian, and European regulatory agencies and may become available in Canada and/or Europe before it is available in the United States.

Sexual Rehabilitation

But what about a woman who has gone without regular sexual relations for long enough that she anticipates real pain if she allows penetration by her partner? Dr. Allen, the wise and witty New York gynecologist who specializes in counseling menopausal women about sexual health, makes a firm declaration on this point: "No woman has to face the choice of giving up sex or enduring painful intercourse."

Most of the women in my survey population characterized as "LLs" with Lowered Libido have totally given up on sex, do not use vaginal estrogen, and rarely use self-stimulation or try introducing novelty into their marriages. And once a woman stops "using it," she is on her way to "losing it."

"After many months of no sex, or no estrogen, a woman's vaginal opening begins to shrink in size, and the lining of the vagina—formerly pink, plump, and juicy tissue when it is estrogenized—grows thinner," says Dr. Allen. Once this tissue is maybe only one cell thick, it often tears when the penis enters. A woman may not be aware of these microscopic tears.

"There's this sandpaper-like feeling when he enters me" is the way women often describe the sensation. Or they feel stinging upon entry of the penis. Or after they have sex, thinking they were lubricated because there is still a watery moistness, they feel stinging when they urinate. That means there has been a tear. If those microscopic tears build up, they easily invite bacteria and infection.

Also, the vaginal tissue stops lubricating the way it did before meno-pause. Dr. Monica Peacocke, a scientist and vaginal specialist in New York, describes the difference between "good lubrication" and "bad lubri-cation": the good kind is the thick and gliding mucus that flows during sexual arousal in women who still have normal estrogen levels or who are using hormone replacement therapy. The "bad lubrication" is thin and watery due to the decreased estrogen level after menopause, and while it may feel like normal moistness, it does not smooth the channel for the penis.

In cases where genital tissue is weakened, it can be made healthy again. But those who don't know they can be treated may resist sexual activity and even masturbation for so long that the anatomical changes will be that much more difficult to reverse. "It can become a vicious cycle," says Dr. Allen, "and then it takes more than estrogen to rehabili-tate the vagina." This vicious cycle can be avoided altogether if a woman knows what to expect.

"Preemptive action is called for if a woman plans to go on having sex," says Dr. Allen, "because once she gets to the Sahara Desert of the vagina, it can take months to get the vaginal tissue back to pink, healthy, and uninfected, and to reestablish the right pH balance. And"—she smiles—"make the desert bloom again." Dr. Allen got permission to tell me about one of her patients who had reached that Sahara point and the two-month program that brought her back to sexual life.

Judith was 50, two years postmenopausal, and not on hormones when she decided to leave her high-wire job as head of corporate com-munications in a large financial firm and move out of New York City. She and her husband, Robert, packed up their three late-life children and moved to a new home in a beautiful Philadelphia suburb. When Judith went in last year for her annual gynecological checkup, Dr. Allen first seated her in her cozy office for a follow-up chat about her life. She asked Judith, as she does all her menopausal patients, "How often are you hav-ing sex?"

Judith looked down and mumbled, "Well, you know, Robert gets up very early and comes home very late. And on the weekends, we're doing the soccer thing."

"So let me get this straight," Dr. Allen replied. "Robert is getting up every morning at five, getting on that train, heading into New York, worried about the day, arriving home at eight o'clock at night, having done the reverse commute. He is supporting a wife who used to work and three children in a lovely, but no doubt costly, suburban home. What is Robert getting out of all of this?"

Judith looked puzzled, but she was accustomed to this doctor's commitment to placing a patient's care in the context of a full life history.

Dr. Allen fixed her X-ray-strength blue eyes on Judith. "Do you still love him?"

"Of course!" Judith said.

"Do you want to remain married to him?"

Judith was surprised that the doctor would even ask such a question.

"Did he used to like sex?"

"Oh, sure!" Judith answered. "We both liked sex. But"—and she paused, as if unsure of how to explain it—"we're just getting older."

Dr. Allen got straight to the point: "Look, I delivered your kids. I know Robert. He's a great-looking guy, and he's in the city sixty hours a week with hot babes. Unless something is wrong with him, sooner or later he's going to get tired of your obligatory sex."

Judith sighed, and then said, in almost a whisper, "Doctor . . . you know . . . it hurts."

"I can fix that!" Dr. Allen proclaimed. "All you had to do is tell me that you were having a little vaginal dryness."

"This is way beyond vaginal dryness. Sometimes I feel like crying."

When Dr. Allen examined Judith, she found that her genital tissue was thin, pale, and dry. Her vaginal opening was very small. And while she was being examined, Judith exhibited signs of secondary vaginismus, a condition where the woman squeezes the muscles around the vaginal opening to close it and avoid pain, or as a barrier to intercourse. It's a reflex.

"Don't worry," Dr. Allen told her. "I'm going to rehabilitate your vagina."

Dr. Allen taught Judith how to use Vagifem by inserting the tiny applicator in the office. Most patients who are already having pain are reluctant to put *anything* into their vagina, and Dr. Allen has found that leading them through it helps assuage any fears. She put Judith on a

Vagifem regimen: every other night for the first two weeks to jump-start the re-estrogenization process, and then twice a week. In a follow-up visit, the gynecologist taught Judith how to exercise the vaginal muscle and to relax it with gentle heat and massage. She also showed her how to use a set of dilators to stretch the opening.

In four weeks, Judith came back to Dr. Allen's office, and her vagina was pronounced cured. But there was still more important work to be done. She needed to rehabilitate the intimacy in their marriage. Dr. Allen suggested that Judith have a talk with Robert. "You need to explain that you had not understood what had happened to your genital tissue, that you had become reluctant to have sex because of pain and didn't understand that you had any other options. You need to tell him that you thought it was just a part of the natural process of growing older. And then," Dr. Allen winked, "I want you to have vaginal intercourse, using a lubricant. You don't have any responsibility for being orgasmic. I just want you to be able to have sex without pain."

Judith came back two weeks later and told Dr. Allen what had happened. "Robert said to me, almost *tearfully,* that he had begun to think that he didn't understand what his life was all about. It had suddenly become his father's life—working to support children and a wife at home, with nothing for him except going out on Saturday night with other local suburbanites, having a few drinks and dinner, and coming home and maybe once a month having sex." There were tears in Judith's eyes now. "I didn't know *any* of that!"

Dr. Allen smiled. Their intimacy rehabilitation was well under way. But the doctor wasn't finished. She herself is a practiced flirt. Pat Allen is also the only woman I know who would wear slingbacks with three-inch heels to wade through New York's winter snow slush just because she's meeting her husband for dinner. "But he hasn't seen me in three days!" she'll say. This attention to the male visual sense is what allows Dr. Allen to keep up her busy medical practice with its late nights and emergencies and to beg off boring country club dinners with her husband's clients if she has a date to see the opera with a girlfriend.

"Here's what I would suggest," she told Judith. "Ask Robert if you can set aside fifteen minutes a week on Saturday mornings for private time. Therapists say this to patients in marriage counseling all the time:

take fifteen minutes and work on your relationship. Do you think he'll do that?"

"Oh, yeah," Judith giggled. "Now that we're having sex again, I think he'd be more than happy to."

"Speaking of," Dr. Allen said. "How'd it go? Any discomfort?"

There was none. In fact, she'd had an orgasm during foreplay. Dr. Allen often suggests foreplay orgasms as a way of further relaxing the vaginal muscles during intercourse. They'd had sex, and it had been comfortable; better than comfortable, it had been intimate, something that had been missing from their relationship for a long time.

"Dr. Allen," Judith said during a later visit. "You saved my marriage."

Better Than Sex

No matter how old we are, we never lose the hunger for a loving touch and emotional closeness. Among women of a certain age, those aspects of a relationship are often more important than the sex, or, at least, the starting point for satisfying sex.

In *As Good as It Gets,* Jack Nicholson, as Melvin the homophobic curmudgeon, bursts into a hotel room and finds his lady love, the waitress Carol, played by Helen Hunt, in bed with their gay traveling companion. "Did you have sex with her?" Melvin demands.

Carol responds, "To hell with sex." She looks hard at Melvin, who ducks her gaze. Then she smiles at her gay friend. "We held each other. It was better than sex. What I need, he gave me great."

As we get older, we don't need more frequent sex, and intercourse may less often be orgasmic, but the mutual caressing, unguarded love talk, playful fantasies, and falling asleep in the spoon position can be more deeply satisfying in terms of emotional intimacy. We never lose the need for touching. We are animals, after all, and when did you ever meet a dog or cat that didn't need petting? If touching is not available by a romantic partner, it's worth it to seek out a good massage therapist. Pets are great touchy-feely companions, and the best ones feel your pain.

Lucy, a California woman with long thick raven-colored hair and a seductive shape, had been single and sexually athletic until her mid-forties.

That's when she started menopause—a sudden jolt to her way of life and libido. When night sweats made her feel as sexy as melted candle wax, she began mainlining tofu and soy. It didn't help much. Her doctor, a practitioner of preventive medicine, told her that soy in quantity is not healthy. Her flashes subsided only after she developed healthy habits such as exercise and began using homeopathic doses of estrone and progesterone. She still loved sex and continued to have it. She was a single woman and she thought of herself as being not much different from the way she was when she was in her twenties.

"I was with a younger man who was very well endowed," she said. "It was wonderful at the beginning, then it started being less comfortable, and by the time I was forty-eight or so, it was like, 'Oh my God, major pain!' "

Like many women, she was fooled into thinking she was still juicy because she lubricated very well when aroused. What she couldn't detect was a thinning of the tissue in the vaginal area. "I kept promising I'd find another gynecologist, but I didn't. And finally, when sex literally became too painful, we split up."

Lucy was in denial that she had reached the stage of menopause. Once she let go of the desperate need to prove her perpetual youthfulness and consulted a gynecologist who recommended using topical estrogen in the vaginal area, it became possible for her to have sex again without pain. As she made the passage into postmenopause, she found herself able to enjoy a sexual partner who is five years older.

"He takes care of me before he takes care of himself," she confides. "I don't have to see him every night. It's better, because now I have time for my work and to go dancing! I wouldn't say my sex drive is what it was before, but I feel it has a more appropriate place in my life at this stage. Instead of feeling desperate to be touched and have sex, now it's just a wonderful outcome of intimacy."

Chapter 13

Seasoned Sex Is in the Mind

*T*he higher seat of desire, for women, is above the neck.

What women need is the right partner, the right context, or the jolting reminder of what attracted them in the first place, and passionate love can bloom again. If it involves a new mate, it exposes a woman to risks and self-discoveries that can be the catalyst to beginning a new phase of life. If it is a revitalized love within an existing marriage, it can fuel the deepest satisfaction as the couple experiences mutual growth.

The most convincing proof that seasoned sex is in the mind comes from postmenopausal women who have been without intimacy for months or years. They may have resigned themselves to thinking that sex is but a memory. Then even an image, or a phone call, can start the juices flowing again. If a woman is bold enough to initiate closer contact with the source of that flicker of desire, it can lead to the most amazing sexual fireworks ever.

A Midlife Sexual Awakening

"I felt like I had dried up in every way—even my genitals had shriveled."

That was how Sheila began her story. A successful woman in a gossipy Texas town, she asked that a pseudonym be used. Like many of the WMDs I interviewed, Sheila's marriage had presented an attractive and socially acceptable shell. Early in their relationship she was able to have multiple orgasms, but by the time she entered midlife, her marriage had become toxic on the inside. "The emotional connection is what counts after fifty," she stated knowingly. "Even if sex can be technically satisfying—i.e., orgasm achieved—without a deeper connection, it is not so satisfying."

Childless, she had gone through menopause at 47 and gradually retreated from all but occasional sex with her husband. "He suffered from premature ejaculation and was always criticizing me for being too slow," she revealed. His selfishness reawakened angers she had repressed from a period of sexual abuse in her childhood. She felt herself shut down sexually and in most other ways. It was a little death.

Obviously, something else of signal importance had happened between that time and our interview. Sheila was now 56 and she looked radiant, with the coloring of a china doll.

"I went through six or seven years of working on myself to get up the courage to leave the marriage," she told me, "and at the same time I was determined to 'fix' it. All the while, I was going through a tremendous personal metamorphosis. But my husband insisted I hadn't changed at all."

Facing the midway point of her fifties, Sheila was appalled at what was happening to her. She gave her husband an ultimatum: if things didn't change by the end of the year, she would leave him. When the year was up, she initiated a separation by sleeping in a separate bedroom. About this time she began talking over the phone to a man with whom she had long felt a mutual attraction. They had been friends as couples, but now he, too, was separated and filing for divorce. They shared the special rawness of being at the start of a frightening passage. They affirmed each other's struggle to give birth to a new self. Her phone friend told Sheila that he could hear the change in her voice, and it excited him.

"Incredible feelings came up." A smile broadened across Sheila's face and her fingers stretched out. "I opened up. Even before we got together, just talking over the phone, I began having spontaneous orgasms."

Sheila's experience highlights the fact that a woman's libido is not a prisoner of age and fluctuations in her hormone levels. Every bit as important for women, if not more important, is the context—the emotional and psychological background tone to one's view of life. When Sheila perceived that she had "shriveled up" in every way, it was because the new self struggling to break out encountered only disdain from her husband. Once that emerging new identity was appreciated by another man, her juices began flowing in every way.

When her divorce was final and Sheila was free to give herself to the love affair, she was astonished at the intensity of feelings that ricocheted through her—from ecstasy to despair. "I'd have orgasm after orgasm after orgasm. And I felt it not only on a physical level but as a spiritual, soulful experience. It's hard to find the words to describe the feelings, including sadness, having wanted it so badly within marriage and finding it in an affair. I used to be so judgmental of friends who had affairs—I would cut them off. It's totally changed my way of thinking about what 'connection' really means. His loving has healed me."

Sheila's affair was destined not to last, but it was the precursor to her seeking professional help in dealing with the residue of her childhood sexual abuse, and moving on with confidence in her desirability as a woman. She was just beginning to recognize that her lover was probably a transitional figure. His wife had a chronic illness, and he couldn't bring himself to leave her. As Sheila told this part of the story, she sounded fragile but determined. "It's extremely painful to give that up," she admitted. "My body has grieved. I hope I'm grieving the old me dying as the new one is coming into being." She was then able to be philosophical: "Losing a relationship like this in the past would have sent me into a cycle of depression. What it's done is to show me that I don't have to hang on to a man to feel strong."

Finders, Keepers

Use it or lose it. Is there a woman who has not heard that famous rubric of the sex researchers Masters and Johnson? Science has demonstrated the organic truth of that statement: women who have regular sex are more easily aroused and make more eager partners. Or, to put it in a nutshell, the more sex they have, the more they want it.

Women whose marriages have gone cold or who are without a steady partner repeat the same complaint: "I can't find anybody to use it *with!*" Many of the respondents to my questionnaire indicate that they are "too shy" to put themselves "out there." Further questions often reveal that they are dismayed by their own hypercritical mental image of their bodies or the imagined ruin in their faces, and they are terrified of the indignity of rejection. Consequently, they are more likely to comfort themselves with overeating, slacking off on exercise, letting themselves spread, dispensing with the effort of coloring their hair or giving themselves home facials, and settling into a wardrobe of boxy blouses and elasticized waistbands. Then, if the fleeting possibility of a fling with the tax man presents itself or an old boyfriend emerges from the nostalgic mists of the past, they have lost the sexual élan to capture the moment.

The women who gravitate to my group interviews are likely to have "lost it" for a while—for months if not years—but to have "found it" again with a Pilot Light Lover or a consciously revitalized marriage. And once they have found it, as the song goes, they may never let it go. So I offer an addendum to the Masters and Johnson rubric:

Finders, keepers.

There is a strong symbiosis between a woman's bodily self-image and her sexual response as she gets older. Women who keep themselves in shape, who discover a good vibrator sooner rather than later, who have a little collection of erotica to keep themselves stimulated when they're without a man, are much more likely to tell me they were ready when the opportunity presented itself.

Another story suggests that even a seasoned woman of 70 who is depressed and suffering from arthritis can revive her *joie de vivre* through the healing powers of sex. Regina is a voluptuous woman with a colorful personality and a penchant for wild love affairs. She has outlived three husbands. Accustomed to being appreciated for her sexiness, her seventieth birthday hit her hard. Alone in a New York apartment and increasingly crabbed in walking or writing by arthritis pain, she descended into depression and sought out a psychiatrist.

"In my bathroom there's a mirror opposite the shower," she told the doctor. "I feel like I walked into the shower at forty-five, came out, looked in the mirror at seventy, and everything was eight inches lower."

Several years passed before she crossed paths with a former lover she hadn't seen for decades. He was now 80, and she was 74. They became impassioned lovers. She made her last visit to the psychiatrist and told him, "Not only is my depression gone, my arthritic pains have disappeared!"

❖   ❖   ❖

Dr. Judith Wallerstein, author of *The Good Marriage,* scoffed at the comment often made by unmarried Seekers among my interviewees: "I don't need a man to define me." "You bet they do," argued the psychologist. "Sexual attractiveness is central to a woman's self-image, and no one develops a self-image alone." The adolescent girl is made aware that she is changing when she's noticed by boys in a new way that is both exciting and frightening. During a woman's twenties, thirties, and early forties, male attention may be expected at parties and even in business situations and becomes part of how she interacts with men. As she moves into the late forties and fifties, gradually, reluctantly, she notices her sexual attractiveness waning in its effect on strangers. Fewer and fewer men give her a second look on the street and at parties. If there are younger women in the room, she needs a well-developed gift for conversation to distract attention from the visual competition.

But an older woman should not write herself off so quickly. The testament to her attractiveness can be convincing if it comes from a loving partner. One of Dr. Wallerstein's subjects described a transcendent moment that restored her deteriorating self-image. This woman, in her fifties, left her marriage for a few weeks and went off to a country hotel with a lover. Once inside the room, they embraced and began hungrily peeling off each other's clothes. As they climbed the steps to the loft bedroom, she noticed a full-length mirror at the top of the stairs and felt a shiver of self-consciousness. Had she surveyed herself, she would surely have seen only the flaws or thought, "Oh my God! I'm looking more and more like my mother!"

Instead, she saw the reflection of her lover's face, behind her. In his eyes was a reverence for her reflection in the mirror. She glowed.

This is one of the reasons that love affairs from years past are so quick to be rekindled, because of what Dr. Wallerstein calls "double vision—holding on to the early idealizations of being in love while realizing that one is growing older and grayer and cannot turn back the

clock." Couples she studied who were in long, good marriages still pre-
served a treasured image of the partner from one of their first encounters. Decades later, the husband can describe the glow around her hair
when they met, or her body in a white bikini. The wife recalls how vulnerable he looked sitting cross-legged on the floor at a meeting for divorced parents, or how he ignored the rain streaming down his face when
they ran into each other's arms after a lover's quarrel. "That double vision," says Wallerstein, "I think is central in maintaining a romantic
relationship."

I have noticed in my interviews that women with a negative body
image in midlife carry around a subjective age that may be older than
their actual years. If they don't think they look sexy, and they don't feel
sexy, they don't put out the signals or scents that attract others like bees
to a flower.

The Botox Generation

But what of women who have a distorted image in the other direction—
who are desperate to believe they are twenty years younger than the im-
poster pictured in their passport? We all have a private, subjective sense
of how old we are. When I ask people in interviews how old they feel, unless they are depressed, the age they give is invariably younger than their
real age. Forty-year-old women and men are most likely to say, "I still sort
of figure I'm twenty-eight." The difference between our real and our subjective age shifts over time, and in people with a healthy self-perception,
the gap probably becomes smaller. If you're a 65-year-old woman and
you feel as though you're 55 or 58, that's natural and adaptive. If your
self-perception is too distant from reality, you are not going to function
very well in the world.

Injectable youth has been seized upon with a vengeance by members
of the Botox Generation. Since the FDA approved Botox in 2002 for the
reduction of frown lines, it has been the fastest-growing cosmetic procedure in the United States. The craze for erasing the folds and creases of
age begins quite young. Almost half of all surgical and nonsurgical cosmetic procedures in 2003 were performed on Americans aged 35 to 50.
The 51-to-64 age group is close behind, accounting for nearly a quarter

of all procedures, of which Botox injection is the most popular. Indeed, some dermatologists buy the botulinum toxin, type A, in bulk and invite patients to "Botox parties." We have all noticed women whose overuse has left their faces frozen in a Stepford wife stare.

Cosmetic fillers last for only about six months. A fling with a younger man can do more to reverse a debilitating self-image and boost a woman's desire and desirability than any Dr. Lookgood's needle. But there is an important caveat: a woman who hangs on at all costs to a young Pilot Light Lover is likely to end up tortured and stripped of self-respect. The most vivid example of this path came from a woman I will call Sydney, who joined one of my group interviews in a western state. I relate it as a cautionary tale.

"The Very Thought of You . . ."

When I first met Sydney, I would never have guessed her age. Tall, trim, and still able to belt her blue work shirt into tight jeans with a big silver-and-turquoise buckle, she is the picture of an ageless sportswoman. Her blue eyes are set deep and flash like cobalt. Her blond hair is still styled like a boarding school girl's: straight and flat with a part.

"I'll be seventy next year."

Gasps from the younger seasoned women gathered around the table for a group discussion on a hilltop patio in the Southwest.

"I can't believe it either." Sydney laughs. "I think of myself as still forty-five. But I have grandchildren from age twenty to two months."

Sydney was widowed at 45. Shockingly widowed. A car crash. "That was in another life," she says, and before we can commiserate, she moves briskly on to the more titillating part of her story. She had moved from Washington, D.C., to a mountain state to forget her loss on the ski slopes. She fell in love with her ski instructor, who was ten years younger. He taught her to live on the wild side and experience a new sexual reality. On hearing this capsule introduction, some of the women in the group expressed envy. Most had grappled with no longer being a babe. Sydney's sexual adventures had apparently allowed her to push her confrontation with the Vanity Crisis to the limit. We were all eager to hear her story and how it had played out.

"Oh, my word!"

That was her expression when she looked down from the chairlift on her way to the top of Sun Valley. Sydney spotted her new ski instructor below, leaning nonchalantly on his poles, and she drank in his beauty. She thought to herself, "He is the handsomest man I've ever seen in my life!" Sydney had flown out to Idaho with her 14-year-old daughter and grown sons to maintain the Christmas family tradition, although all were still in shock from her husband's death only six months before.

Her expression, "Oh, my word!," serves as a mantra describing her social class and the imprint of her generation. She is clearly a thorough-bred with high cheekbones and a long, lanky frame that suggests she was born with her feet in silver stirrups. Her pre–World War II puritan up-bringing denied her any thought of an independent life. She did what was expected of her gender and class. "I always was the perfect older child," she tells us. "I did all the just right things, graduated cum laude from Vassar, and never had a teenage rebellion." She produced four beau-tiful children, kept immaculate homes, and looked forward to their an-nual family Christmas ski trip to the wilds of Idaho.

Sydney had never been on her own.

In the year before the sudden loss of her husband, both of her parents had died. The three losses so close together left her utterly adrift. In the presence of her handsome young ski instructor, she felt herself sliding back in time, from the frozen widow to the unfinished girl—caught up in silly, selfish, lusty, devil-may-care rebelliousness.

Within several more months, Sydney was back at Sun Valley, this time with a woman friend. "I called him up when I got there in March, and I knew I wasn't going just for a ski lesson. Amazing, for someone so conservative. I was suddenly so much sexually freer." The other draw was their athletic connection. "He taught me how to really ski," she says. "It was magical. I never stopped being with him after that."

Her lover wanted to move away from his ex-wife to another ski resort and become a writer. Sydney had enough inherited money to finance his fantasy. The hardest part was introducing him to all her East Coast friends; they were appalled, and some dropped away. Sydney's former mother-in-law refused to come for Christmas unless the pair stopped "living in sin." So after their first year together, Sydney married her ski instructor. It was a reckless decision that she would come to regret.

Sydney knew when she married him that her lover had two young children and was a self-professed recovering alcoholic, although he still smoked pot rather regularly. "But I was so head over heels in love with this guy, I ignored the warning signs," she admits. She encouraged him to write a book and then financed its vanity publication. When it won an award, she felt justified. She was exhilarated by their adventure trips together; every other year they went trekking in the Himalayan mountains of Nepal. For the first ten years of marriage to her ski boy, time and cares were pleasantly suspended. Sydney was able to perpetuate the fantasy that she was still young.

But as she moved into her sixties, the gap between her physical stamina and that of her younger husband widened. Many of their favorite daredevil pursuits became difficult or impossible for her. The meanest and most startling of penalties was in their sex life.

"It started when I was about fifty-eight or sixty," she says, "the drop-off in my desire. I went to three different women gynecologists. One said, 'Oh, I'll fix your ailing libido in a minute.' She put me on a higher dose of hormones, but I still wasn't having much response." A psychiatrist diagnosed her as depressed and gave her Prozac, which seemed further to dampen her desire. She began faking her orgasms. But the real dampener on her desire was the simmering resentment that threatened to break through her denial of the obvious: that she was allowing herself to be exploited and treated badly.

They saw a couples' therapist, who told her husband, "Sydney's getting older. You must understand that she can't keep up with all the things you do." That infuriated Sydney. She worked even harder at keeping up. But a few years later, they went to Kathmandu with the goal of trekking up eighteen thousand feet to the base camp of the third-highest mountain in the world. A few thousand feet before reaching the camp, Sydney's endurance gave out. She was 65.

Age and financial realities had finally caught up with her fantasy of agelessness. Sydney was addicted to an Adonis figure who was depleting not only her resources but her physical and psychological stamina. He started drinking again. When he wasn't teaching skiing in the winter, he was hiking and biking with his guy friends while she sat home depressed. A young woman joined his hiking group. In Sydney's eyes she was "a homely jock girl," so she didn't worry. Although her inheritance was dwindling by now to a dangerous level, she made one last attempt to revive their marriage. She sank $350,000 of principal into building an idyllic getaway for them on the coast of Mexico, imagining herself and her ski boy walking naked on their private beach, swimming like dolphins, and recapturing the passion of their early love. He rewarded her by secretly spending a week in the new house with his jock girlfriend.

"It shook me to the core that a girl who looked like that could take my husband from me. It was humiliating." Her fury was focused only on the wound to her vanity and self-image.

Now comes the kicker to her story.

Over Thanksgiving vacation that year, Sydney took her children to the house in Mexico and stayed on for three weeks. She shed fifteen pounds and whittled her body down to a taut 122, which began to make her feel attractive again. She read books that stimulated her sense of herself as still seductive, including a biography of Edna St. Vincent Millay, which described the writer's torrid experiences. She remained, however, stubbornly resistant to changing in any other than these superficial ways.

"I'd never been thrown over before," she says, "and at sixty-eight, I didn't plan on doing my life over."

Her husband called her and said he still loved her. She asked if he loved the jock girl. Yes, he said. She challenged the idea that one could love two people, but in truth, the sexual rivalry excited her. After their conversation, Sydney walked the beach until her imagination swept her backward: "I kept 'seeing' him all over the beach, swimming in the ocean. In my fantasies, we'd just finished this house, and it was just for us. I knew that would never be, but my fantasies turned me on and I began to feel sexually hungry again."

She invited her husband to join her at the beach house. In preparation for winning him back, she ordered sex toys from the Internet and lace teddies from Victoria's Secret and bought long satin pants and sexy tops, which she wore without lingerie. On their first night there together, they slipped naked into the hot tub and moved on to the shower, the bed, the floor. Her narcissistic need to feel young again was well satisfied, for the moment. "I was feeling good about my body, I was feeling sexy," she says. "It was the best sex ever. Which proves to me," she emphasizes, "that for women, sex is all in the head."

❖   ❖   ❖

But it's not quite so simple.

Sydney's lost libido was not about hormones. Nor was it about the man, whom her imagination allowed her to convert from a cad into a prince. That recurrent fantasy was fueled by her desperate need to retain the idealized image of herself she had once seen reflected in her ski boy's eyes—the image that allowed her to believe she was still 45. So long as she dissolved herself into the romantic passion, she didn't have to change or grow or face her losses. Or did she?

"We can't expect a lover to do the work we haven't done for ourselves," says the San Francisco psychologist Dr. Melanie Horn. "When we try to use a relationship to defend against painful feelings, we get stuck." Sydney had escaped facing her traumatic grief by retreating to an earlier stage that she had never completed—adolescence, with its urge for rebellion—and that retreat had allowed her to postpone for the next twenty years the necessity to evolve into full adulthood. She had enough money to insulate herself inside a fantasy marriage, but she paid dearly for the sexual passion of those years—in financial terms, in the falling away of lifelong friends, in the ebbing of self-respect. Ultimately, the blatant evidence that she was being exploited curdled her sex drive, and she slid into depression. Her resistance to rebuilding her life in her sixties only postponed the reckoning.

The longer a necessary passage is postponed, the harder it will be when it is finally, unavoidably, confronted.

In the months after her ravishing week of sexual reconciliation with her husband, it became obvious that they were not connected in any important way except the physical. When they went out together, it looked as if they were going to two different parties—he sported a tattoo and earrings and dressed in shorts and Birkenstocks; Sydney always dressed up her jeans with silk tops and elegant ethnic jewelry. She became increasingly resentful of the inequity in their financial situation, and her complaints, he told her, made him feel emasculated. At last she was able to make the break from the man she'd used to keep from facing herself and valuing her own real worth.

Slowly, Sydney is adjusting to life among the liveliest of her own peers. She spends time with her golf group and her ski group, but she is also looking for a more sustaining, nonsexual passion so she can use her time and money to benefit those less fortunate in her community. Sydney was nearly 71 when she was able to acknowledge, "In the end, sex wasn't enough."

Chapter 14

Spicing Up Midlife Sex

One key reason that the majority of divorces taking place after age 40 today are initiated by women, I have surmised, is sexual frustration. I am amazed at the number of women who tell me they didn't realize until after their midlife divorce that they'd never had an orgasm with their husbands. Why? Because many husbands still don't know, or perhaps care about, the anatomical fact that Kinsey proved: that for a woman to reach orgasm, she needs clitoral stimulation.

The Reverend Billy Graham condemned Dr. Kinsey's "secret agents" for interviewing women about intimate details of their lives and vouchsafed that "their lives are not typical of the Christian women of America." That's quite the opposite of what I found out when I plunged deep into the Bible Belt to interview women. Even as the abstinence movement is spreading among conservative educators of high school kids around the country, a lot of sex education among adults these days is going on at sex toy parties. And it's mostly married women who are the avid consumers of sex toys. Women invite their friends to home parties where saleswomen give demonstrations of sex aids along with tips and titillating patter. Husbands who wouldn't give their wives a nickel for another Tupperware party—"We don't need any more plastic!"—send them off to these sex-ed sessions with the blessing of credit cards.

Eastern Arkansas is cotton-picking country, where everyone goes to church on Sunday and keeps their drinking, gambling, and fooling around under wraps. In my interviews with women there, as in many other parts of the country, I found a persistent gulf between public "moral values" and private sexual behavior.

Passion in the Bible Belt

Linda Brewer is being pulled over, again. She steers her Cadillac Escalade over to the side of the road, rolls down her window, and calmly waits. This kind of thing happens to her all the time, especially here in Sheridan, the tiny Arkansas town—population 3,872—where she grew up, raised her daughters, coached softball, and ran a sporting goods store. She watches the cop approach her in her rearview mirror. She hasn't met this one, yet. He saunters up to her driver's side window, pulling off his sunglasses and using them to gesture to her rear bumper. "Ma'am," he says, "what does the FUNLADY do?"

"Well," says Linda in her throaty voice, giving a little wink, "it's not Tupperware."

It was Linda's second husband who bought her the FUNLADY vanity plates five years ago after she became a Passion Parties counselor. Unlike most counselors, who visit hostesses' houses with suitcases full of sex toys and marital aids, Linda runs what she calls an "open house" out of her own home, a block from the largest church in her county. It is essentially a sex toy store with one huge difference: no men slouch through shadowed hallways picking out the latest addition to their porn collection. Linda's sex toys are all discreetly concealed, each in its own labeled drawer. And her clientele is made up exclusively of women—churchgoing women.

One of the pastors of the church was forever stopping at her home and trying to persuade her to come to church with him. She would beg off, "Brother, you know I can't come." He would promise to set her up in the pulpit with him, hoping to assure her acceptance in the community. But after a nasty little incident in Dallas, Texas, Linda is afraid to proselytize in public. In 2004, a Passion Parties counselor was arrested by two undercover narcotics officers after they purchased two vibrators from her in a sting operation. Headlines branded the former elementary school teacher the "Infamous Dildo Saleswoman." Under an archaic county regulation, she faced a year in prison and $4,000 fine, until a judge dismissed the case against her "to avoid wasting county resources."

"So the pastor refers clients to me at home," says Linda proudly. "They stop by directly from church." After Linda closes her open house at seven P.M. on Sundays, the calls start coming in: "Linda, can I come at eight, when there's nobody else around?" The FUNLADY is quite content to go along with the game. Despite her tiny customer base in a rural southern town, she consistently ranks as the company's number one in personal sales.

Like so many of the company's top employees, Linda started out with a miserably deprived marriage and no money of her own. She was lured to the company when she saw other Passion Parties counselors driving around in fancy cars and flashing diamond jewelry. "In the twenty-five years of my first marriage—and I've never admitted this to anybody in the world—I had maybe two orgasms," she says. "I thought an orgasm was something you read about in a book. For nine years I slept on the couch. I would wake up in tears. I'd go to see a gynecologist and he'd say to me, 'Linda, I think you're just sexually deprived.' He suggested masturbation. Well, you know what we were taught down here—if a girl does that, hair grows on the back of her hands."

Attending her first Passion Party, she got so excited about the prospect of becoming a saleswoman herself, she purchased $180 worth of items. She went home and told her first husband, "I can do this, I know I can."

He replied, according to Linda, "Who in the hell are you gonna sell that shit to?" She answered, "I don't know, but I'm gonna find them." And she's still finding them. The starter kit for a saleswoman cost $1,200. Linda scratched up $500 and borrowed the remainder from her son-in-law. Shortly after starting as a Passion Parties counselor, she met her "fantasy man," her present husband, who she says opened up new worlds for her.

Like most of Passion Parties' senior counselors who qualify for Diamond Level status, Linda has since become an evangelist for the power of sexual pleasure to transform a woman's life and elevate marriage to ecstasy—of the kind she claims to enjoy with her second husband.

"That's why I can relate so well to my clients. They come to me with the same frustrations I used to have. I talk with them about how to work things out. Then I start them off with a silver bullet [a battery-operated pocket vibrator], and they find such a release, they bond with me like they do with their doctor."

I asked Linda, "What is the most valuable thing you have learned about older women and sex?"

"How wonderful it is to have an orgasm, whether you're with your partner or by yourself. Sexual satisfaction can change your life," she answered.

"Have you seen that?" I asked.

"Seen it? I've lived it."

The First Lady of Passion

Passion Parties today is indeed the Tupperware Party of the new millennium. A privately owned national company estimated to do about $20 million worth of business in a year, its sales staff is composed of almost three thousand "counselors" who pay to be part- or full-time franchise operators and, in turn, induct other women as salespeople on whose proceeds they get a commission.

The street-smart sales genius behind this exploding business is C. J. Haynes, otherwise known as the First Lady of Passion. She is in her mid-sixties and looks like what she is, a grandmother, albeit one who is a sharp dresser with an even sharper tongue. As the top-ranking grosser in the company, she and her group sold $5 million of merchandise in 2004. Her territory is Arkansas, Tennessee, and Mississippi—among the deepest states of the Deep South. (More recently, sales have exploded in California, Washington state, Wisconsin, New York, Arizona, Texas, Missouri, and Ohio.)

The major consumers of vibrators, says C.J., are not cosmopolitan women frustrated by their single, sex-in-the-city lives; her prime customers are married southern women. She educates them about their biology in a subtle and witty way—right down to the specific location of the clitoris and the "G spot." She brings to her sessions the same evangelical zeal as Kinsey; her goal is to make American marriages more vibrant. When I tell people C.J.'s story, their first question is, "Why are Passion Parties such a big hit in the *South*?"

"What other entertainment do they have?" asks C.J., in a whiskey-tinged voice that always sounds slightly conspiratorial. "Women down here are repressed. Ninety percent of the jobs they get here are factory jobs for $5 to $7.50 an hour. There's no place to buy sex toys in Arkansas. They come to my parties to see the toys and learn how to use them. They also come for the camaraderie, and to show off how much money their vibrators cost."

When C.J. picked me up in one of her three Mercedes with her pearl-handled revolver in the cup holder, I must have looked startled. C.J. laughed. "Honey, no way I'm going to leave outta here without my protection."

When C.J. first went into this business, she was working for a company in Tennessee. She commuted between there and Memphis, where her husband was employed. C.J. was in her forties and looking for a side gig as a tax write-off. Her daughter had been to a sex toy party and called to say, "Mom, you're going to love this!" C.J. ordered the kit on approval. "There was stuff in there that I did not know what to do with. Here I was, a grown woman, with kids who were grown, and I've got this twenty-two-year-old secretary telling me, 'Well, don't you know? That's a cock ring.' " C.J. was both shocked and underwhelmed. "I thought, 'Hmm . . . Tupperware . . . sex items . . . let's give it a year.' "

She organized her first party and booked four more parties before it was over. After six months, her parties were bringing in a significant amount of money. She kept track of her receipts and sent them in to her tax man. He called her up and jokingly said, "If you're selling pot, C.J., I'm not sure we're supposed to be claiming tax write-offs."

She began recruiting other women as distributors, women who were raising kids by themselves and keeping just ahead of their house payments. C.J. would tell them, "You don't need your crummy nine-to-five. You can make more money doing this, and do it around your own schedule." The job that had started as a tax write-off began to take on the fervor of a mission: "I was getting girls off welfare." C.J. was doing so well, she jumped into a higher income bracket. At that point, she quit her job and moved to Memphis. She soon became the first in the company to bring in $10,000 a month.

When she went to her husband's banker in Memphis to open a business account, he asked what kind of business it was. "Oh, no, I'm sorry," he said. "We can't let you do that down here."

"Why not?"

"We just don't do that down here."

C.J. laughed in his face. "Then where is Tennessee getting all these babies? Importing 'em from Mississippi?"

This was all twenty years ago, and C.J. was full of stories about the cussing and dissing she endured to get around the antiquated social and legal norms of the Old South. Before she was permitted to do any shows in Mississippi, she had to stage a show for a judge and his wife and friends. In Memphis, she had to do a mock show for the city council. "I've been thrown out of hotels, but you know what scared me the most?" She gives a deep, gurgly laugh. "I almost shot a woman's husband. She was the sweetest woman you ever saw. She had fifteen of her friends over, and they were buying like you would not believe. I'm starting to pack up my suitcases, and I hear this banging and cussing going on upstairs. I went back in the house, and her husband's got her up against the wall. He was drunk. He threw some racist remark at me and shouted, 'Get your ass out of my house!' " C.J. looked up at him and said, "You touch her and I'll blow your blankety-blank brains out!" That's why she always packs her pearl-handled gun.

◆   ◆   ◆

We drive from Memphis across the state line into the swampy former rice paddies of eastern Arkansas. In what seems like the middle of nowhere, a subdivision of modest bungalows appears. As C.J. unloads her trunks of toys, the hostess strides out in jeans and buzz cut, a Pall Mall cigarette dangling from her mouth, her teenage daughter behind her. The hostess is a hairdresser who hears all the secrets of the women in town.

Inside her living room, fifteen women are splayed in overstuffed lounge chairs wearing shorts and flip-flops that display lots of hot pink, well-shaped toenails. Smoke hangs heavy in the air. Everyone snacks unabashedly from paper plates sagging with dips and fried food. Most of the women have grandchildren, and one is a widow of only three weeks. The living room is filled with china cherubs and fake flowers, an antique jukebox, and a massive TV that takes up one wall. When C.J. is ready to begin her presentation, she asks, "Does the TV turn off?" Someone answers, "I've never seen it off."

With the zeal of a tent preacher, C.J. extols the virtues of Lickety Lube, Passion Powder, and the Little Beaver Finger Vibe. The women hold out their arms obediently to be sprayed, gelled, and tickled, concentrating on the various sensations they're supposed to be feeling. They follow her commandments religiously, a room full of straight-A sex disciples.

"A lot of women in the South are sick of having religion stuffed down their throats," she has told me. "Our women use sex as a tool because sex is so male-dominated here. And these women want pleasure for themselves."

In response to a stimulating cream, a traditional-looking lady asks innocently, "Whose man will like this?" The married hostess answers: "Who cares what he likes? It's about us."

Giggles around the room.

When C.J. demonstrates a waterproof vibrator, the hostess exclaims that it will be great to use in her backyard pool. "The cop living behind me is gonna get a whole lotta show this summer!"

"That's my momma," says her daughter.

C.J. winds up by demonstrating vibrators in the shape of ball bearings and butterflies, hummingbirds, dolphins, and rabbits. When she retires to the back room to hold private consultations with each of the guests and take their orders, the shy women mark their order sheets covertly. The bolder ones stand up and shout, "Save some for the rest of us!"

Chapter 15

Sex and the Seasoned Marriage

*S*ummertime. Elegant dinner party. Round tables, each with eight guests seated within easy earshot of one another. One couple, seated opposite, is having a *Who's Afraid of Virginia Woolf?* moment. The other couples make an effort to ignore their acidic barbs. Suddenly the wife's voice pierces the polite hum of party conversation.

"My husband and I haven't had sex for eighteen months!"

Heads turn away. Gaping silence. Nervous clatter of utensils. The toxic moment has almost passed when the husband recovers enough ego to reply.

"What about last Tuesday?"

The wife, dripping contempt: "You call that sex?"

"All the guests suddenly mumbled excuses and, within five minutes, fled," the hostess told me the next day. From the look of horror in many eyes, it was obvious to her that other couples were identifying all too vividly with this overt display of a middle-aged marriage that has become a living death.

❖　　❖　　❖

What keeps two people together through the surprises and setbacks of middle life? Once the children are launched, any marriage undergoes a tremendous shift. You must decide if you are in the marriage now because you *want* to be, not because you *have* to be. You may decide you still want to be because he's a good man—not perfect, but good. Or because he's been a good companion in the past, or because you have a shared dream for the future, or because your history together is precious and you hope to build on it with new adventures and joy in your grandchildren-to-come.

There are four pillars I have observed that seem to hold up long and solid marriages:

- A love deeply enough felt that each of you cares for the other as much as for yourself.
- A negotiable power balance. By that I mean that both partners have developed the ability to compromise and to give in, as well as the strength to hold firm when it really matters.
- A vested interest in each other, in your children and family life, in your shared faith or belief system, and in your shared history. When you can be proud of what you have produced and are passing on together, it confers worth on your individual life as well.
- A sense of humor. An appreciation of the absurd allows us to hit the bumps of life with a little more bounce. Professional matchmakers say that a consistent requirement of both women and men looking for a potential partner is a sense of humor.

But just as important as these pillars is a powerful destressor that helps a couple ride out the inevitable rough patches: making love. It is in the surrender to shared passion that many of the tensions we cannot talk about find release and even resolution.

Some of the best sex is among couples who have been together for a long time. Surprised? Of course you are. That is not the message suggested in Victoria's Secret ads or any movie you see, but it's true. There is a fundamental misunderstanding that good sex doesn't happen inside a marriage. In fact, it is the emollient of a good marriage.

Inevitably, of course, a long-term monogamous relationship becomes stale without work and planning from both partners. Not just commitment, which can be dutiful and dull. Sex at this point has to be a much more conscious activity because in the middle and later years libido is reduced for both the male and female. You plan sex because you value it, not because your libido is driving you the way it did when you were 25. And when you plan sexual encounters, lovemaking can actually be that much more exciting, because you own it. It's not happening by chance because one or the other is turned on now and then. You may decide to engage in more fantasy or more foreplay to get the juices going, or to find an inexpensive getaway that can become your private love nest. It's the conscious buy-in—both partners being willing to make an investment of time and resources in their love life—that creates a channel for fun, pleasure, and deepening love.

Recapturing the ardor takes a bit of education and pleasant work, and many of us are not capable of getting there on our own. Sex therapists teach couples who are in trouble how to revive their sexual connection in a conscious way. If the couple has had good sex in the past but the marriage is in transition, somebody has to be able to step back, take a look at the situation objectively, and say, "Do I want to throw the baby out with the bathwater?"

An Erotic Workout

The latest area of bodily enhancement sought out by the spa set is the sex-ed workshop. The first program of its kind was developed at the Canyon Ranch in Tucson, Arizona, by Dr. Lana Holstein and her husband, Dr. David Taylor, both medical doctors. Open only to married or committed couples, the program has evolved into a four-day retreat, offered for a hefty price, at the exclusive Miraval fitness resort, also in Tucson. This unique workshop attracts mainly couples in their forties, fifties, and sixties who are ready to focus on their intimate relationship in a new way. People in second marriages who have passed through the infatuation phase are also well represented, ready to take a prophylactic approach to extending their sexual connection. (For those without the luxury of spending $6,800 for a long weekend in a lavish spa, Drs. Holstein and Taylor wrote the book *Your Long Erotic Weekend*.)

Dr. Holstein teaches couples that what they really want to work toward is "the soul connection." What I found surprising is the therapist's conviction that couples find their soul connection by planning for *consistent, reliable, repeatable sex.* It sounds like the opposite of the oft-touted spontaneity and novelty. Yet Dr. Holstein maintains that reliability and planning are the keys to "the persistence of passion."

The erotic weekend begins with group sessions, where couples don't have to say a word; they are taught sexual biology and counseled in how to pleasure each other. During the afternoons, in the privacy of their rooms, they work on "homework" assignments. "The important thing is to start experiencing fully giving, and fully receiving, sex," says Dr. Holstein. "That means being willing to let go of your old wounds and angers and being really open to your partner."

Inhibiting dynamics are often exposed. "A lot of women are very good at giving, and yet when we assign them the homework of just receiving, being pleasured, with no intercourse, a woman often feels vulnerable and apprehensive," says the doctor. "She's so used to thinking she's supposed to be doing him. And when she's just receiving, she can't take control." When the man is assigned the role of giver, he is not just expected to touch her genitals; he's also in charge of setting up the room, choosing the music, orchestrating the whole event. It relieves the woman of having to be in charge, but also robs her of controlling the agenda, which may hold her back from enjoying the occasion. She may find excuses not to do the assignment—the couple gets into a big fight, she storms off, and an interesting dynamic is revealed.

The next day the men are pleasured by their women. Now it's the men's turn to reveal their hang-ups. "He's accustomed to being in charge and to orchestrating how she touches him—now do this, no, over here—and that is not just receiving," explains Dr. Holstein. "If he were touching himself, he might do it a little differently, but what we want the couple to experience is not getting to orgasm in 6.5 seconds, but allowing themselves to give, or be given to, and experience something much more profound." This is what the counselors call "the soul connection."

This is the antithesis of seeking only novelty to spice up the midlife marriage. Recognizing that as we are all pedaling at a much faster pace, with a cell phone held to one ear and a PDA at hand, it requires a more conscious commitment to carve out time for true intimacy with our partners. Where do we find true intimacy? It is found at that point of attachment where your hearts beat as one, when love is transmitted through murmurs and caresses, and you *know* and *are known.* That can open the door to the secret place where you are both truly "at home"—a place to which, with practice, you know you can return, because you know the techniques that open that door.

Shall We Dance?

This is not to say that novelty is to be sneezed at; it's another spice to add to a seasoned marriage. I discovered some of those spices in a most unlikely place—at a health ranch during a women-only week.

It was in the dance classes: Women still in the final blaze of youth, women whose bodies had lost their shape, women who had never dared be on display in tights in a coed gym, women of an age assumed to be asexual—all shapes and ages of women came out. And there, with no male spectators, we could express ourselves—our graceful, or wounded, or angry, or erotic selves—in a nonthreatening environment.

The Afrcan Dance class required a hip wrap—why? As women in vivid sarongs thrust their pelvic girdles with unaccustomed zeal, I began to understand the transformative effect of a simple hip wrap. We moved across the dance floor in a half-crouch, waving our arms and pounding our heels to the beat of an authentic African drum. Our teacher was a four-foot-eleven spitfire whose fluid body and bodacious pigtails made her look like a candidate for carding at any club.

"I'm forty-seven," Connie Bennett told us proudly, "and I'm hell-bent on going to the big five-oh!"

In salsa class, my partner had a full but shapely figure and seventeen great-grandchildren. She moved like a dream. When Ruth Anderson told me she was 74, I couldn't believe it. "Dancing is my outlet," she confided. "I don't get to dance at home. I've been married twice, but both husbands have two left feet." Ruth had never before given herself a vacation alone, and she was reveling in it. It was plain that her adored, left-footed husband was going to benefit handsomely from the renewed zest she would bring home from this all-women's week.

NIA was another class I had never tried; its mysterious name made me suspect it was some kind of cult. When I learned that it was a non-impact aerobics technique that combines multicultural movements from ethnic, modern, and jazz dance with the forceful movements of martial arts, I decided to try it.

It was another revelation. Shifting from the flowing moves of a swan dance to the swivel of Cuban-motion hips to the brute blocks and kicks of karate allowed for a full range of emotional expression. When the class was over, I noticed one of the guests swabbing tears from her cheeks.

"For me, being in such a regimented, highly structured life and job, it was such a total release," sniffed Meg Schuler. A vivacious brunette, she had come to the ranch to celebrate reaching her fiftieth year. "But I feel like I'm thirty-five," she said. "I'm a very happy person. I have a wonderful husband and I'm fortunate to have a wonderful life. But with a high-level job as a senior vice president of a national company, life is also incredibly stressful." She works seventy to eighty hours a week and has had multiple pregnancies but no children.

"This dance class let me be free—back to the totally uninhibited person I used to be and knew still existed inside," she continued. "I'm going home to my husband and tell him, Harry, I've got to do the things that keep the child alive! It's so much a part of who I am. When I'm walking by the pool in our backyard, and I feel like jumping in, I don't care if I have all my clothes on, I'll just jump in! And if I want to sing out loud, I'll do so."

The NIA instructor easily empathized with Meg's tearful release. Marilyn Tradewell has seen countless numbers of her women students react the same way after a session of this therapeutic movement— including herself.

A slip of a woman with china-white skin and a hood of jet-black hair, Marilyn is easily taken for 45, tops. She is 60. So slender, so limber—but she has not escaped self-doubt or depression. On the contrary, it is in overcoming those tendencies in her Second Adulthood that she has become stronger and more spiritual. Over lunch, she told me her story.

In her forties, a divorced Marilyn had faced an inconsolable loss. Her only child, a son then 20, was hit by a drunken driver and massively brain damaged. Doctors pronounced him as good as dead. The hospital called her to ask for consent to harvest her son's organs. Marilyn charged to the hospital and said, "I do *not* consent. He will not die."

The force of that moment changed her whole approach to life. You feel it in her class when she demonstrates the martial arts moves that are part of NIA choreography. "It teaches women to draw firm boundaries."

After living at the hospital with her son for two years, she made the decision to take him home. Doctors told her he would never walk, talk, or think. Her love and intuition allowed her to reject those predictions as well as perilous surgeries. For the last seventeen years she has dedicated herself to finding ways to bring her son back through natural movement.

"I'm pretty stoic," Marilyn told me. "So the grief didn't really hit me until five years ago." Her son's boyhood friends were graduating from college, marrying, having baby number one, then number two. Marilyn would meet with their mothers and listen to them talk nonstop about their grandkids. She was in her mid-fifties without a prayer of ever having such a joy. "It really hit me—the fear that instead of becoming a grandmother, down the line I would have to think of a group home for my son. I think I did have a depression. It showed up in immune system problems. I developed an allergy to makeup; I had digestive problems and felt pain in my ovaries. Then I lost my hair. I wasn't on any medication. It was my own system that was toxic."

Marilyn had remarried after her son's accident. Her second husband adopted the brain-damaged boy and has supported Marilyn's efforts. But she was so good at appearing to be the strong, stoic one, teaching Pilates and taking care of everyone else, she couldn't get her husband to understand that there was a deeply wounded mother grieving underneath. That accumulated emotional pain had translated into a destructive force working inside her body. It was only recognized when Marilyn visited a gastroenterologist in Los Angeles who also happened to be a shaman and a healer. The doctor did not have to examine Marilyn. She just looked straight at her and said, "You have a right to live."

Marilyn realized, "I was leaving my life."

Around the same time she found NIA. It was a moving meditation, through which she discovered her self and her center. Her fatigue evaporated. Age seemed to have no claim on her. She accepted that she had a right to live with full expression and feeling. Once Marilyn felt focused, she found a new passion and purpose in becoming credentialed as an NIA instructor.

"Instead of leaving my life," she said, "I am dancing through life."

◆   ◆   ◆

One night at the ranch I gave a talk on *Sex and the Seasoned Woman.* The response was telling. Meg Schuler bounded over to me. "I took in everything you said. I'm going home and telling my husband, 'Get ready, Harry, we're starting over again!' "

The next morning, in circuit training class, I was approached by one of the most attractive women among all the guests. A Texas beauty with long blond hair, a ski-jump nose, and slim, tanned limbs, Janie DeGuerin looked like the last person to be worried about her sex appeal. I figured her for early forties.

"I'm worried I'm one of your 'Lowered Libidos,' " she blurted out. "I love my husband and he loves me, and we've always had a great sex life. But now"—she wrinkled her lovely nose—"the libido is less. He feels guilty that it's his heart medication. I feel guilty that it's my hormones. I'm fifty-six, and he's fifty-four and—"

I stopped her. "You're fifty-six?" I wanted to reassure her that yes, the libido does lessen as we move into our fifties and sixties, but it's nobody's fault, it's nothing to be ashamed of. Other Lowered Libidos I'd interviewed had given up on sex, or resigned themselves to just grin and bear it. But she was here, tuning up. As long as Janie and her husband loved to be together, the two of them could invent their own choreography of love.

I was yet to discover the best spice of all. There I was, on a sultry August afternoon, doing tai chi. While my class was somberly rocking from one foot to the other, eyes closed, something far more primitive was going on next door. The women who came out of that gym were all laughing like naughty girls and humming in a decidedly burlesque manner. "What class did *you* take?" I asked.

"Strip dancing."

I made it my business to get to that gym the next day. Let the tai chi people levitate to higher consciousness; I wanted to get down with the girls who strip-danced.

The teacher, Demetrius, a young African-American man with an imp-ish smile, told us right off the bat, "Strip off your usual identity. Throw it away. Decide who you're going to be for the next hour. Is it going to be Beyoncé? Or J.Lo? Gypsy Rose Lee? Whoever . . ." He pulled on a wig. "I'm Ginger."

He told us to pick out a long, diaphanous scarf in one lurid color or another and then strike an aggressively sexy pose. Each of us stood be-hind a folding metal chair. "Okay, you're in the VIP room. There's a man in your chair. You're going to do a chair dance." He put on the music from the movie sound track of *Moulin Rouge*.

At five-foot-four, with enough years on me to rate a senior movie dis-count, I'm never going to move like Nicole Kidman, and neither, pre-sumably, are you. But I could take on the character of Roxie, the moll with moxie in the musical *Chicago*. There were women in the class who looked well beyond the age of performers. But it didn't matter one bit. Nobody was looking at any of us—we only had eyes for Demetrius, and ourselves.

As each of us put one hand on the back of a chair, Demetrius counted down, "Five-six-seven-eight," and we were off strutting a Janet Jackson walk around the chair, then hanging off the back of it, grinding our hips to one side, then the other, and then down in a hammocky swivel.

Well, every woman in the room began to shake her booty, dangle her ornaments, and toss her head in a slave-to-love swing, all the while strok-ing her chair as if Brad Pitt were sitting right there. With the scarves wrapped around our fannies or swirling around our necks, we shame-lessly stroked our hands up and down our inner thighs, and over our tum-mies and breasts, flinging our arms high in the air with squeals worthy of Marilyn Monroe. Before you knew it, we were on our backs, kicking our legs, and pulling up with a long erotic moan—"AAAgggghhhhmmmmmm-mmm . . ." You have never seen so many middle-aged women vamping.

Next to me, I caught a glimpse of the sylphlike NIA instructor. Mari-lyn was switching her head from side to side and throwing her long black hair in a slave-to-love motion that was decidedly different from her usual swan dancing. Meg was on the other side, producing moans of lust. Be-hind me was a tall, strikingly slim woman who had the hip rotations ex-actly right. I later learned that Jennice Fuentes was raised in Puerto

Rico, so she had the inbred advantage of Latin-motion hips. Most of us had been raised doing strict ballet or Martha Graham modern. And there were some women behind those chairs in their seventies and over.

Ruth Anderson, my salsa partner with the seventeen great-grandchildren, was flinging her scarf with delicious abandon as she snaked around her chair. Next to her was a petite African-American woman who moved with the sultriness of a jaguar stretching in the sun. She was not young.

"What brought you to strip class?" I later asked Anne Patterson.

"Well, at eighty years old, I figure that anything new is exciting, and I want to try it!" Her eyes flashed. "And I might just use it the next time I see a young man who interests me."

Demetrius told us that stripping practice is good for releasing your inner goddess. I whispered to Marilyn, "It feels more like a release for your inner harlot." She nodded. As we polished our routine, Demetrius stopped the music and announced with mock-seriousness: "Okay, we're performing at five o'clock this afternoon—makeup, costumes. What are you going to call yourselves?"

"The Harlettes!"

Before my next talk, I asked a few of my sister novice strippers to do a demonstration with me as the windup. We had ten minutes to rehearse before our audience gathered. Demetrius showed up with the music five minutes before. When I finished my talk on how to pursue a more passionate life, and announced, "Showtime!," the Harlettes leapt to their feet, wrapped themselves in scarves, and struck their chosen poses. I introduced them.

"Desirée." Meg cocked her leg and dropped her chin.

"Lolita." Jennice did a backbend while batting her eyes.

"Star." Marilyn jutted a hip and stroked her black hair.

The women guests stood and clapped us through the routine. We were—may I say?—great. Our little demo had the effect of a power surge that spread throughout the ranch. The Texas blond who feared losing libido hired Demetrius to give another chair-dance class for those who had missed the first one. She called her husband to tell him about it. The next day he sent her flowers.

On our final night, the ranch prepared a beautiful poolside dinner.

Everyone put on makeup and real clothes for the first time in a week. With the first drizzle of wine and the sudden impudence of bongos played by a Mexican band, we all loosened up. Half the crowd rose to its feet, squeezed onto a tiny wooden platform, and burst out in an all-female bacchanalia of interpretive dancing under the moon. Not quite howling, but close.

Meg made good on her promise to be true to her inner child. Her face crimson from exertion but wreathed in smiles, she led a conga line around the pool. And around again. Until the mood struck her to lead everyone to dive in. Fully clothed. Screaming with delight.

Swinging in Silicone Valley South

In southern California, the body beautiful is worshiped and slavishly worked for, and God forbid one's eyes should sag or one's chin droop. "It's like Silicone Valley South down here, and I don't mean computer chips," quipped a glamorous lecturer in a workshop I attended on business management. The lecturer looked to be in her early fifties, slender and stately, with a carefully colored hood of chestnut hair that curled under her chin. Her name would be recognized as that of one of the top women business owners in the country; I'll call her Betsey. In the testosterone-enriched environment of high-tech software firms, she holds her own as a president. Betsey looked every inch the confident, successful, attractive model of a seasoned woman, dressed to perfection in authentic Chanel and, what's more, ringed with a sizable diamond attesting to her long-running marriage.

Behind the public face, however, I found a woman torn apart by inner conflict. She is, in fact, 61 years old, and her husband is a few years older. For the past seven years, they have frequented a private club in Hollywood that rents out a movie set on Saturday nights. At a cost of $150 to $200 for the evening, members are invited to change into scanty garb, usually Speedo briefs for the men and sexy lingerie for the women. They then dance with strangers to hard rock and drift off into one of many nooks and crannies to play out their sexual fantasies. The patrons—all couples, no homosexuals—use pseudonyms, pay in cash, and are well protected by security guards.

"This whole scenario is supposed to be sexually exciting, but what's been happening is it's made me less sexual and less interested in sex," Betsey confides.

The couple was turned on to the secret swinging subculture by old friends who had just returned, ecstatic, from a swingers' convention. The chief proselytizer and his wife are highly visible sacred cows in their community. Betsey's husband was very interested. To Betsey, it was a crazy, even repulsive idea. But she likes to think of herself as a curious person; hadn't she always wanted to try skydiving? And who was it who had always dissuaded her? Her husband.

She tagged along with him to the next swingers' convention. "It was like going along to a football game that you don't really want to go to," she says, "where everybody's screaming and yelling and getting into it and having a wonderful time and you're sitting there thinking, 'God, this is so stupid, all they do is run these balls back and forth!' " She laughs. Then just as abruptly, her eyes close tightly against an ooze of tears.

"I've had such terrible anguish about going to this swingers' club. I've told my husband several times, 'I'm not going to do this again. I can't stand it. Why don't *you* just go?' But he says it wouldn't be any fun for him if I wasn't there." Her voice is breathy, high, childlike. Although she speaks frankly, there is an undertone of meekness and embarrassment.

The greatest anxiety in the back of Betsey's mind is attached to the number 15. That was the number of years her first marriage lasted, before it was shattered by evidence of her husband's gross infidelities. "One of my secret goals is to have this marriage last longer than my prior marriage," she says in a near-whisper, "and we're at that critical turning point—the fifteenth year." She sees this husband as her best friend and soulmate. They are both high achievers, and he accepts her for the high-powered executive she is, without jockeying for position.

Sometimes she laughs at herself, as if she attends these parties for some sociological purpose and can stand back and say, "Huh, isn't this *fascinating.*" The truth is, she admits, the swingers' club brings back all her earliest girlhood fears of inadequacy: "Are my breasts big enough? Will men like me?" Then suddenly she shows a flash of adult anger: "Can you imagine? Here I am, a full-grown adult with grandchildren, a very successful career, visibility, a pillar of the community—can you imagine what this would do to my reputation if my friends knew?"

When I suggest that it sounds as if she has been giving in to subtle coercion, Betsey confesses a deeper cause of her anguish: "It is not what I would call outright coercion. It's that I want to please him."

So many married women can relate to this. Putting their husband's pleasure before their own is a natural feminine instinct, but it often detracts from their own sexual satisfaction, which, in turn, can make sex less pleasurable for their husbands. Probably the single greatest obstacle to becoming a truly seasoned woman—or man—is to violate one's own values or moral code. Betsey's story is a vivid illustration of the price to be paid. For all her power and self-confidence in the professional domain, she has forfeited any power in her marriage in exchange for emotional security. As a result, in her business life she's at the top of her game, while in her personal life she's back at the bottom of that pit of self-doubts where she started as an awkward adolescent.

Betsey's quandary brings to mind the sex scandal that took down the career of a good-looking Republican Senate candidate, Jack Ryan of Illinois. His wife, Jeri, had graduated from being a National Merit Scholar to being a beauty queen to being Seven of Nine, the babe poured into an intergalactic catsuit on TV's *Star Trek: Voyager,* a mechanical male fantasy who wrestled with trying to become human and sexual. When her politician husband began to insist on frequenting sex clubs, Jeri went along for a while, she alleges. One night, she says, when her husband took her to a club with whips on the wall and cages hanging from the ceiling, she broke down and cried, becoming physically ill. Finally, she sued for divorce. Court papers described the sordid marital contract Jeri claims her husband had tried to enforce. He denies her allegations.

In my view, what swingers' clubs appeal to is our fear of entering into the mature years. They offer eager participants the illusion of a return to early-adolescent sex. For the reluctant spouse, they represent a theft of dignity and self-respect.

The Transformative Affair

Helen Gurley Brown's voice is still low and seductively breathy and her comments are as baldly candid as when she reinvented the formula for *Cosmo*. Helen is now 83 and still married to her only husband, David Brown, who is 89. By all measures, they appear to enjoy a well-seasoned marriage. They both still go to their offices and do what they love every day; he makes movies and produces plays; she critiques the foreign editions of *Cosmo* that are implanting her formula all over the globe, including in two Muslim countries. Helen is sympathetic to women whose marriages have deteriorated to the point where the couple functions as roommates, or where they are permanently separated.

"After fifty, you may be by yourself, but there are ways to start up again," she says. "Even masturbation works. The challenge, because it's more fun to be with somebody than by yourself, is to find somebody to be your companion. I recommended in my book *The Late Show* that you borrow somebody's husband if necessary."

That suggestion produced a furious outcry from some of Helen's married women friends. She hastened to assure them, "Not *your* husband, but there are married men who aren't having much sex in their lives. Why not take a needy married man to a nice hotel and have a rendezvous with him, *just for the purposes of sex?*"

Given that Helen is an old friend, it was uncomfortable to put to her the obvious question: Had she made an arrangement with her husband to allow for this practice?

Helen lets go a deep chortle. "My husband is off limits. And even at our age, we do have a sex life. So I'm not loaning him out, and I don't have to borrow anybody. David had been married twice before, and this time he finally got it right. We didn't marry until I was in my late thirties, so our sex life was consummated late and it's continued to go on. Even so, it helps if you go away on romantic trips and plan rendezvous—that's what people do when they're younger."

Helen is able to take her husband on trips to exotic corners of the world for openings of new *Cosmo* editions. Last year alone, they were in Russia, China, Serbia, Bulgaria, and Bosnia. "When you are in another city and in a glamorous hotel, that is conducive to sex," she says. "You think, hey, let's don't let this go to waste." Helen is characteristically blunt: "An orgasm is an orgasm, it doesn't matter how long it takes to get there."

While Helen's husband-borrowing solution seems dicey for all parties, she is on to something. An affair can jolt people out of a dead marriage, or rein them back in, once they realize what they stand to lose. Dr. Ethel Person, the Columbia University psychiatrist who writes so perceptively about romantic love, observes that some of the most transforming and positive love affairs are in fact adulterous.

"Some unhappily married people use the reassurance they can derive from a happier, or ego-enhancing, affair to enable them to leave what has become a stultifying marriage—even when they cannot marry the lover who makes such a passage possible," she says. She gives illustrations of women who slip, almost unawares, into a passionate relationship with a man who cannot offer a long-term resolution to their unhappiness. But when they do subsequently remarry, some years later, that relationship may prove to be much more fulfilling and happy, in part because they have developed enough confidence to be less neurotically dependent. "While one may take exception to such relationships on religious or moral grounds," writes Dr. Person, "from the perspective of the participants rather than from that of the observers, these love affairs provide the sense of meaning, transcendence, immediacy of experience, and transformation that are the essence of any reciprocated love."

A wise psychologist in Berkeley, California, Dr. Hilda Kessler, tells the story of a patient who was in her mid-fifties when, for the first time in her marriage to a fine man, she was swept up in an intense sexual affair. "We talked in therapy about how the affair was highly narcissistic—an adolescent recapitulation. One night she had a vivid dream in which she saw the things she cherished most all disintegrate. She realized the affair would ruin her husband, her children, and herself, and she decided to end it. When she put the affair aside, she used that sublimated energy to become passionate about painting and became very involved in community arts. She has since done some fabulously creative things." The consequences for her marriage were also beneficial: she was able to re-create their union on much more egalitarian grounds. It was fortunate that this woman was in therapy at the time and could consciously look at what she was doing, even as she was doing it. If she hadn't been aware of why she was exploring her sexuality outside the marriage, she might have broken the vessel that holds the meaning of her life.

"I've seen a lot of women do that," says Dr. Kessler. "Women who insist their marriage is terrible and they have to get out—in some cases, they haven't done the work of growing themselves, or growing the marriage. The grass looks greener. If they get out and the grass isn't greener after all, then they're in a pickle."

A woman who busts out of her marriage in midlife needs to ask herself: *What are you trying to achieve? Is this about some piece of leftover development? Is this about proving to yourself, or to your ex, that you are still desirable? Is this an escape from the need to find a new dream to enliven your Second Adulthood?* Most psychotherapists draw a clear distinction between a sexual affair and a love affair. The purely sexual affair may remain a secret, and if the woman is still in love with her husband, it might turn out to be beneficial to both of them.

There are other, nonsexual ways to revitalize a long-running marriage. One of the more thoughtful responses I received was from a 55-year-old woman in California:

"This is one of the tough times for us in our 31-year marriage—menopause for me, retirement and 'midlife crisis' for him. But we'll make it through. Here are a couple of things we are doing to refresh our partnership: We dance. The other thing we do is entertain in our home. Generally, we have dinner parties for eight about once a month. We invite people we know but who frequently do not know one another. We plan and cook the meal in coordination with one another and enjoy interesting conversation around the table. The pleasure often carries over for days with us."

The Last Word

Dr. Pat Allen, the New York gynecologist, is now in training to become a sex therapy counselor. Some of her women patients in long-term, monogamous relationships confess to the doctor that they have no interest in sex and engage in it only because "he wants it, and I do it as little as possible." Dr. Allen will start by asking if he has been a decent husband and they have enjoyed good sex in the past. If the answer is yes, the doctor will likely observe that the marriage is just in transition, and the couple doesn't quite know what part of the puzzle is missing. "The fact that you are willing to give him obligatory sex is just not good enough," she often points out. "Your husband is probably feeling your rejection, your anger, your unhappiness." She acknowledges that keeping a marriage alive by keeping the sexual connection alive is a choice that requires a change of attitude and some hard work. She advises a patient to start by paying attention to her husband in a sensitive and romantic way, pointing out that men respond better to action than to talk, talk, talk. Dr. Allen's advice, based on her long clinical experience with midlife women, is meant to shock and awe:

"Stop talking and start lovemaking."

Part III

*Learning to Be Alone
with Your New Self*

*A*s a percentage of our adult life, the amount of time we spend being married is shrinking. Why? Because we continue to live longer, marry later, exit marriage more quickly, and increasingly choose to cohabit before marriage, in between marriages, and as an alternative to marriage. Consequently, an entirely new ratio between married life and singlehood is becoming the norm. According to research by the National Marriage Project at Rutgers University:

> Most Americans will spend more years in singlehood throughout their adult lifespan than in a continuous marriage.

This is especially true for women, who live longer, and normally outlive men by an average of five and a half years. So it behooves us to learn sooner rather than later how to do more than survive on our own. We need to learn how to *thrive* on our own.

"I have friends who have been single their entire lives, and I'm struck by the differences between them and women married for long stretches," says Barbara Dafoe Whitehead, co-director of the Rutgers National Marriage Project. "The never-married women have learned how to have very interesting, full lives on their own. For married women who become single, it can be really hard to gain that level of social confidence if you haven't been practicing for a long time, especially at an age when you probably aren't building social networks at your workplace."

If practice is the key, better to rehearse before it's actually required. The wife of a hotel manager who had channeled all her love and attention into her three children admitted in a group interview in Las Vegas that she was still suffering from the loneliness of her emptied nest. Her children were well into their twenties. "I'm now able to go four or five days without talking to them on the phone," she said proudly. She is in her early fifties. I asked, "Do you feel a new self, an identity of your own, coming into being now?" Her eyes glazed over. She said, "I was always taught to blend into my husband."

Stories like this highlight why married women need to learn how to be alone and build an independent identity as much as, if not more than, single women. The single or divorced woman is forced to explore how to fill her life with stimulation and purpose. It is all too easy for a woman with a demanding husband and overscheduled children to lose track of what once made her feel unique.

If you want to carve out a seasoned woman, get rid of everything that isn't a seasoned woman. Open your eyes to your actual feelings, drives, dreams, desires, and, just as important, your dislikes. Take back the power and authority you have too easily granted to others, and begin looking for the genius within yourself. Let go of the dreams that weren't realized in your earlier life, and let yourself re-dream. Then you will be ready to reestablish your life around a new, or renewed, passion—that is the secret. And if you are religious, you may forge your new dream with divine guidance.

In this book, you have come across a number of stories of women who have spent a good year or more learning to be alone and fostering a new identity. Peggy, the professor who lost her husband to prostate cancer, regained her "wild hair," or fun-loving nature, by daring herself to try new things alone. Sandy, the Texas woman who risked the death of her marriage, used a separation from her husband to take a faith walk, and found a new spiritual foundation on which their marriage was resurrected. Other women went back to school and, finding a new focus once they completed a degree, committed to supporting themselves.

As women, most of us are so habituated to organizing, planning, making lists we never complete—operating the switches of that incredibly complex machine known as family life—that we allow little or no time to nourish the spirit within. If we are to fulfill our higher role as "carriers of the culture," we must begin in midlife to cultivate the habit of caring for our own soul. This will probably necessitate a bold separation of some sort from the status quo of daily activities.

But I don't have time to take a hiatus! you'll say. You have too many people depending on you—a husband who lapses into despond when you're away, an ailing mom or dad in Florida, a floundering child who can't seem to take hold in adulthood, your staff or patients or students or co-workers, and on and on. Many of us will resist taking a time-out to do an internal exploration until we run into a life accident that forces us to stop and take stock. Such periods, when it feels as though time has almost stopped, are actually deep, internal growing periods. If we can give ourselves to the process and come to accept that everything serves—even divorce or the death of a loved one—and vow to learn from it, not to be embittered or defeated by it, but to grow stronger from it, then we have committed to growing into a seasoned woman. We have something to build on.

Taking a Time-Out

"I ran away from home at fifty-one."

Joan Anderson makes her announcement without shame. She is a plucky postmenopausal author who escaped the resentment of so many academic wives by taking a moratorium from her marriage to spend a year by herself on Cape Cod. Feeling that her life had slipped completely off track, she had an important question to ponder: "Now that my traditional roles are finished, what am I meant to do with the rest of my life?"

She left her very busy professor husband behind in New York and took up solitary residence on the Cape in the off-season. Taking a bunch of calendars and old journals with her, she tried to reconstruct what passages she had started or finished in recent years. She couldn't think of one. When she looked over her calendars and inside her journals, the record was all about producing, coordinating, organizing. "We are the event planners and family ritual makers, the mothers and the grandmothers," Joan says. "We're all on autopilot—we need to learn to treasure the moments."

There comes a point when we have to say, "Time to stop." Time to retrieve the raw materials of the person you were.

Joan spent a lot of time walking the beach. She would observe the

shore birds marking a softly heaving, translucent waterline; an hour
later, when she walked back over that same stretch, the shape might be
jagged and the colors deep and the tempo of the dance between water and
sand much more agitated—everything would be different. The thought
came to her: "We are all as unfinished as the shoreline of a beach."

One day, walking along the wintry-fogged beach, she saw a mysterious figure in a hooded cape standing on a jetty. The French lieutenant's
woman? No, it was actually Joan Erikson, the wife of the famed professor and author Erik Erikson, who pioneered the study of adult development. Joan, too, was taking time for herself on the Cape, while her
husband continued to be lionized.

A major issue to be negotiated in a marriage at this stage is the equa-
tion between autonomy and dependence: What does the couple do separately, what do they do together? Joan Erikson herself used to complain
that her husband would ask her, "Where are you going?" She told friends,
"I didn't mind telling him, but I didn't want him to ask."

The two voluntary "academic widows" became good friends and
counseled each other on how to use their solitary time for wise growth.
Joan Anderson wrote a trilogy about her experiences—*A Year by the
Sea: Thoughts of an Unfinished Woman; An Unfinished Marriage;* and *A
Walk on the Beach: Tales of Wisdom from an Unconventional Woman*—
and now lectures on the subject. She acknowledges that few women
would want to take off a year, but what about a week's retreat? Or one
weekend a month for six months? You will read in the next section about
new retreat and revitalization centers that provide for this time alone.

Being solitary for too long is not healthy, of course. And most
women who are alone in middle or later life will miss having a partner to
hold them at vulnerable times, such as when a business deal goes sour, or
her dog dies, or a mammogram turns up questionable results. Science
tells us that we need physical stimulation and a loving touch, not just
when we're infants but all through adulthood and into old age—even if
it's from an animal. Lauren Bacall, the actress best known for being
"Bogey's baby," has lived most of her adult life alone. Now 80 and still
fully active in theater and films, she never goes anywhere without her
dog.

It's never too late to practice being alone. At a party held in Santa Fe for couples who are still married to the same spouse after fifty years, I was astonished to learn that not one of the wives had ever spent any time living alone—not in seventy-five years. In their era, people married early and once, and the rest of life was two-by-two on the ark. One charming Danish-born woman, Anne-Lise Cohen, still beautiful and flirty at 76, had dared to spend a week away from her handsome husband while she was studying for certification exams to become a psychoanalyst. That little taste had given her an appetite for another period of solitude. She made a confession to the group: "Last year, for my seventy-fifth birthday, I gave myself a week's vacation on an island off the coast of Maine—alone!"

"What was it like?" the other women demanded to know, as eagerly as if they were inquiring about an exotic voyage.

"I haven't taken it yet."

Smiling Singles

Being older and single used to conjure up the stereotypical image of a cranky crone whose loneliness and physical complaints were an albatross hung around the necks of her adult children. But contemporary older women have information and resources to prolong their healthy years. They can easily acquire the knowledge to maintain strong bones and extend their flexibility (whether they use it or not is another question). They *should* know how to boost their energy by supplementing the vitamins and minerals that might otherwise be siphoned off by the reduced metabolism that often leaves people over 50 anemic. And should they choose, they have the option of literally freezing the clock with cosmetic interventions. So today, being older and single and still physically strong challenges a woman to expand her horizons and learn how to entertain *herself.*

Here is the truly new phenomenon that I came across, empirically, in my interviews and online research: seasoned women who are single are *not* necessarily unhappy with their lot. *Roget's Thesaurus* has no synonym for such women, offering only the words "spinster, spinstress, old maid, maiden lady, bachelor girl, single girl, lone woman, spouseless, celibate"—all of which carry negative connotations. Many *un*married women over 50 are not looking for another spouse, having had their fill of husband care. They say the same thing over and over: "I don't want to cater." Lovers, yes; many enjoy lovers. Or they move on to commit to live-in life mates or enjoy intermittent intimate friends or traveling companions or sports partners. But a good many cherish their hard-won independence and have learned, or are learning, how to fashion a full life outside marriage.

Sally Denton, a journalist and author in Santa Fe, New Mexico, is typically outspoken on this point. Twice divorced and just giving birth, at the age of 50, to her fourth book, *Faith and Betrayal,* Sally still has three kids at home. "I frankly prefer the company of my sons to any man I've met since my divorce," she says. "My ideal relationship would be committed, but we live in separate houses, keep separate bank accounts, sleep together, hike together, hold hands together in the movies—all the good parts—but we don't get wrapped up in the man-woman, husband-wife, dirty-socks situation."

Grace, a Latina woman who joined in the group interview in Berkeley, had a much bigger cultural gulf to cross in learning to be alone than a feisty feminist like Sally. Grace was raised within a strict Mexican Catholic culture that dictated she stay in her marriage no matter what. She waited out the marriage until her two boys went away to college and she was financially secure in a professional career in northern California. By now in her fifties, she laughingly describes herself as fully "colonized." She has blonded hair and caramel-colored skin, obviously takes good care of herself, and seems planted, stable, an earthy woman.

Divorce was less traumatic for her than she had anticipated. But she hadn't figured on the ache of aloneness. "While you have your children with you, you go to their baseball practices and school events," she said. "Once they go off to college, you find yourself alone. That's a wonderful feeling for a while. As soon as my boys left, I didn't all of a sudden say, 'Oh my God, what am I going to do this Saturday?' "

Grace had her work, which she loved. She is a well-paid, respected hospital director who meets many new people as she circulates among medical centers. "But when I came home, I would think, 'Okay, I can just sit here and read a book and never leave this room, or do I want to try that restaurant that people have been talking about? Why should being alone stop me from doing that?' "

Grace held everyone's attention as she marked the "slow steps" by which she had learned to be comfortable doing things alone. All the other women in the group murmured their identification with her feelings about the "first time."

"I brought a book and sat at a table, opposite an empty chair, and throughout the entire meal I felt people were looking at me, wondering why I was alone, thinking there must be something wrong. Then I realized, no, it's not me; it's them. I actually enjoyed the dinner. It was kind of cool, being out on my own. So you go out and do it again. Little steps. Going to the movies for the eight o'clock show. You see a lot of people with dates, but you go anyway because you want to see that film. And you're glad you did. Then I discovered that in most restaurants, you can sit at the bar. If you go early, it's not date time. People start talking to you, or you start a conversation, and it doesn't feel like you're eating alone. One night, chatting about food started off a nice dating relationship. I didn't feel like I was being picked up. It was very natural. So you don't have to be desperate about going out and looking for men. It will happen. And when it happens naturally, those relationships have been the most satisfying."

Serial Marriage: The New Norm

Women now in their forties and fifties are also statistically much more likely to remarry after getting divorced than were women of previous generations.

"The rise in divorce also means that a higher percentage of people in the more recent cohorts are able to marry twice in their lives," observes Martin O'Connell, senior research analyst at the Census Bureau. The average length of first marriages, for women, is almost eight years. (It's the seven-year itch, plus one. That last one is the year after the woman has emotionally left the marriage and before she actually shuts the door.) Second marriages for women, if they end in divorce, endure even less time—a little more than six years. Added together, that's a married life span of only fourteen years for those who choose two serial mates and disengage from both of them.

It is hardly surprising that after one or more divorces, women in mid-life are by far more gun-shy about remarriage than their male counter-parts. Over half of the women aged 40 to 79 in the AARP study said that, after divorce, they were either certain they did not want to be legally bound to a mate again (43%) or were reluctant to remarry (13%). The men were much more anxious to go back to the married state, presumably because it holds more advantages and less peril for them. Only 33 per-cent of the divorced men were turned off to the idea of remarriage.

The *choice* of singlehood over remarriage is reflected in some of the hundreds of e-mails I have received on the subject from women 50 and over. Here is an example:

I married my best (male) friend 15 yrs older who had a major heart attack 2 years later. No more sex, but I was faithful 'til he died of stroke 18 yrs later. Now, at 55–56 I am experiencing the freedom and confidence to be *me* like never before. I have a very healthy, romantic & actively sexual relationship with a slightly older man. It doesn't matter how long it lasts as long as it's good while it lasts. [Good means] being open and honest, mutual re-spect, each having a crazy sense of humor and being willing to be spontaneous with our lives in all senses. I don't need a "deep com-mitment" but having great sex with anybody just for the sake of having sex—no matter how good the "act" is—doesn't work for me now.

The common thread here is that women are freer than ever to choose the conditions of their Second Adulthood. Just as more are choosing to divorce on the brink of midlife or choosing not to remarry, so those who decide to stay with a long-running marriage *choose* to do so more often—recommitting to the relationship rather than simply drifting along for want of a way out.

Chapter 16

Designing Your New Single Life

period of alone time is almost essential to get to know your new self. It's rather like the way those of us who live in the Northeast feel when we come out of a long winter. Shedding our heavy overcoats and mufflers and boots to walk around on the first balmy spring days, we feel the freeness of having the sun tickle our skin and we move about in a sort of exhilarated trance.

Luisa, for instance, was known to her friends as a serious, shy, solidly goal-oriented woman. She was a planner and organizer who had been married twice, risen to senior vice president of a $2 billion company in Atlanta, and engineered her daughter's acceptance to Harvard. But within her circumscribed universe, she had always had a certain itch.

She wanted to go dancing.

Neither of her husbands had had the slightest interest. It had hardly seemed weighty enough a desire to be called a dream, but the yearning did not disappear, even after her second divorce.

"The first thing I wanted to do was take ballroom dancing," she told me. "I had never done partner dancing. When I grew up, all we did was freestyle dancing."

Why not? That was the new litmus test by which she was beginning to measure her life decisions. She chuckled at the absurdity of it, why so many women wait so long to explore their own dreams. It was such a simple thing—going to a professional studio to learn to dance—but the changes it wrought in Luisa's mood and outlook on life were stunning.

The music called something raw and urgent out of this introverted woman. Before she knew it, her hips were rotating to the infectious rhythms of salsa. Her rather large, broad-shouldered, awkward body lightened up once she learned to waltz. She tried swing and laughed at herself skidding around the floor in sneakers like a bobby-soxer. On Friday nights, the studio invited students to an open dance night where they could dress up and practice dancing with one another, but she couldn't face attending. Suppose nobody asked her to dance? It took Luisa six months to get up the courage to go by herself, not looking for a man, just to enjoy dancing.

"I had learned a new skill, I felt good about myself, it improved my self-confidence and gave me the ability to socialize," she understands in retrospect. She met a new man through the dance classes and began living with him. Without recognizing the repeat of her pattern, she slipped into an emotionally dependent role and remained there until they broke up four years later.

It was only after Luisa crossed the great divide into her Second Adulthood, at age 56, that she began, for the first time, experiencing the freedom of being a single woman not living with a man. After months of watching the tango class, like a child whose nose is pressed against the glass, she got up the nerve to try American tango. She quickly surmised that tango dancers are a world unto themselves. She was never going to pass for Jennifer Lopez in *Shall We Dance?*, but she didn't let that stop her from moving on to the Argentine tango class. She kept hearing that crowd talk about B.A. (Buenos Aires, to the uninitiated), the sophisticated Argentine city to which they made pilgrimages to worship at the shrine of the tango. She felt, finally, that such a trip was within her sights. "Now that my parents were in their eighties and my daughter was in graduate school and I was recovered from my last relationship, I was ready to do something for myself."

She accelerated her tango lessons and hooked up with another woman from the dance studio. They took Spanish at Berlitz and found a bed-and-breakfast in B.A. called Tango House, which was dirt cheap in summer—the Argentine winter.

She lived and breathed tango for a week, and it was a ball. Every night local people mixed with the guests and took a tango lesson at the bed-

and-breakfast. The action in Buenos Aires doesn't start before eleven P.M., so after dinner, the guests would be directed to the best *milonga,* one of the many dance places that offer a mix of mambo, ballroom, and tango. Luisa didn't expect to attract a partner. Argentines don't suffer amateur American tango wannabes gladly. There is a ritual: The man makes eye contact with a woman he would like to try partnering. If she returns his eye contact, that leads to a dance. It's a seduction that favors the man. If the woman turns him down, no one knows.

Roberto made eye contact. He wasn't exactly an expert dancer, but he was very charming and intelligent, an engineer who spoke perfect English. He was also divorced and happened to have children living in Atlanta. She danced with him every night. She had never been so self-indulgent or allowed herself to be so free. "I loved everything about it, and I couldn't wait to go back."

She and Roberto were lovers that week, but she decided in the end that she was not in love with him. "That's not why I was there. I didn't want to wake up every morning with another person that I had to accommodate, or make a plan with, or be back for at a certain time in the evening. It's so easy to fall into a pattern of somebody else's expectations." But she and Roberto had become fast friends, and he promised to visit her in Atlanta.

When her feet touched the ground again back in the States, Luisa felt rather like the exotic artifact that a tourist brings back to remind herself of a life-altering trip. Luisa didn't want to lose the lusty woman she had found inside herself in Argentina.

She toyed with leaving her job. Pragmatism led her to ask instead for a leave of absence. "I was perfectly willing to take the chance that my boss would say that I didn't need to come back. I found myself having to explain to my friends that I was doing all of this from a very positive place. I wasn't running away from my life. The whole influence of Argentina does something to people. It's the balmy weather, the friendliness of the people—even if you don't speak the language well—it's the music, the amazing canopy of purple jacaranda trees above all the streets, and it's inexpensive."

When Luisa was ready to try out her new bicultural life, Roberto took her around B.A. to find a small rental apartment. "For three months

I had a life of not setting an alarm. I'd get up in the morning, go out on the balcony to stretch and have my coffee, take my dog to the park, then I'd head downtown to take a Spanish lesson, and then go on to tango lessons." Although she and Roberto saw each other frequently, she found herself bold enough to walk into *milongas* alone at night. "I did more dancing with Argentines than anyone thought would happen. I learned to live more in the moment."

She planned to go back to B.A. the following spring and look at real estate, buy a little apartment, and eventually set herself up so she can divide her time between her rather rigid, goal-oriented routines in Atlanta and her fluid, languorous life in Argentina. "Finally, in my life, I know what I like. I like cities, and I like dancing. I can't afford to give up my working life entirely, and I need the cultural stimulation of being in Atlanta. But why not make a dual life between America and South America?"

Like all master plans, this one could not take into account the unexpected. Luisa had newfound poise and a figure now whittled by dancing to a sinuous muscularity, accentuated by her new evening uniform of leather skirts, slinky tops, and tango shoes. It was not surprising that she met a man in Atlanta with whom she felt a strong chemistry. He, too, was entering the free space of his sixties, preparing to retire as a school psychologist, and hot to take her on his Harley for a weeklong cycling adventure out West.

Why not? she said. But no strings.

"I'm in the most detached relationship I've ever been in," she told me after the Harley trip, "which is very different for me, and wonderful. Instead of managing my life around the relationship, I just see him when we're in the same city. We might go out to different clubs on a Friday night, or maybe meet up later."

How did you meet him? I asked. She smiled.

"Dancing."

Same-Sex Design

Santa Fe, New Mexico, is a magnet for seasoned women. Women who paint, write, design jewelry, or run one of the many arts and crafts galleries that line Santa Fe's Canyon Drive are drawn to the stark beauty and spiritual energy that have attracted nonconformists to this mecca in the high desert for the last hundred years. The endless sky is a moving mural of colors and portents. There is a feminine quality to the place: every structure has the bulging curves of a woman's hips, since all the homes and stores are one-story, Mexican adobe style, sans straight lines and right angles. Even outside the historic district, where the newer vacation and retirement homes huddle in the hills like soft wombs, the ubiquitous colors are baby's room hues of pink or rose trimmed in blue. The layout of the town is also curvilinear, with the main drag in the meandering shape of a horseshoe, dictating that the only way to get a grasp of direction is by using one's intuitive sense.

Mai first felt the magnetism of Santa Fe when she drove through New Mexico in the mid-Seventies on her way to do graduate work at Stanford University. But for an exuberant woman then in her twenties, Santa Fe was too remote, too solitary. And once she married, had a child, and moved to New York City, the shimmer of Santa Fe vanished in the complexities of love, work, and mothering.

Astonishing changes overtook Mai in her forties. She was divorced at 40. A few years later, to her surprise, never having anticipated a shift in sexual orientation, she fell in love with another woman. She was in command of her own successful wholesale jewelry business. On the cusp of 50, she sent her only child off to college. But it was the internal passage she had been making through her forties that prepared her for the dramatic act of tearing up her old life and starting over.

She and her partner visited Santa Fe together. Mai found herself waxing poetic about how the earth there speaks to you whether you care to listen or not: "Everything is so present—the sky, the clouds, the rain, the quality of dryness . . ." She laughs at her loss of words appropriate to describe the throb of spiritual comfort she felt in this place. She and her partner also found Santa Fe to be full of artistic women, both straight and gay, who form a powerful community. "Back East I felt tolerated," she says, "but here I felt truly appreciated."

It was only the third day of their vacation when Mai and her partner, a documentary film maker, attended an open house just for fun. It was a sprawling adobe with red rock surfaces and a surround of snow-speckled mountains. The *pièce de résistance* was a large studio with windows on four sides and a deck overlooking a high desert garden. Mai heard herself making an offer. It was accepted. "Oh my gosh," she thought, "I guess I'm moving."

Both women were creatively energized by breaking with the East and settling into such a starkly different environment. After a few years, the excitement of collaborating on the decor of the house, dividing space in the studio, and each finding acceptance in her own artistic community died down. They had hoped to find a new calling together, but when that didn't happen, they agreed on an amicable parting.

"Getting ourselves out here was a large part of that relationship," Mai notes in retrospect. "Once settled here, the mission was over."

Six months into Mai's solitary life, she invited me to visit her at home. Having heard her story at an earlier group discussion, I was expecting to find her sad but stoic. She greeted me with a brilliant smile, her gray-blond hair spiked like the fronds of a sea anemone, her full face flushed with the color of an artist interrupted in the midst of intensely pleasurable work. She took me straight up to her sunlit studio, the place where she truly lives. As she moved about in loose black trousers and a woven vest over a pleasantly rounded body, she spoke with reverence about the semiprecious stones and glass beads that sparkled from hundreds of small containers. Each one had a story. There were antique Chinese jade pieces that she had picked up on her travels, Tibetan relics brought to her by friends, some beads so tiny and delicate it was impossible to imagine how they could be strung with the naked eye. Mai introduced me to the Mexican woman who helps her. They often find the stringing process similar to meditation. But Mai's days are not just loosey-goosey artistic swoons. She is also highly disciplined about her work and takes her health seriously. As we talked, she was busy selecting the unique pieces she would take to New York the next day to display at a trade show. From this miniature world, she turned her attention to the mountain that soared just outside one of her windows. "That's where I hike every morning," she said.

How was it living here by herself? I asked when we sat down for coffee.

"I'm really enjoying my solitude," she mused. "It's the first time in my life that I'm living alone." In fact, she wasn't quite alone; she had rented space in her sprawling home to a writer at one end and an artist at the other. Her tenants had their own kitchens, but she liked being in the presence of their artistic energy and sharing ideas with them. "I'm really living in community," she said, "but I'm not interested in a bonding relationship at this point." This surprised her.

A few days before, Mai had had her astrological chart done. The supposedly reassuring analysis had dismayed her. The reader told her that she would have another close love relationship. Normally, one would be pleased, but Mai had walked out thinking, "No, I'm not ready. I really am ready to have a relationship with myself."

Her lesbian partner had played the role of the Pilot Light Lover. Mai's Romantic Renaissance had lasted nearly ten years, but now she was moving on to the next phase in the arc of pursuing the passionate life. She spoke thoughtfully: "I think it's about a spiritual connection with myself and with the world around me. Even though I'm carrying a heavy heart, it feels like I could jump off a mountain and soar. There's something exhilarating about not being in a relationship with all the give-and-take that requires, and exploring what that means for myself. That's not to say that no one will ever pull my heartstrings again. But sitting where I am right now, I feel this is a gift that I've never had before. And it comes from the fact that I'm on the other side of fifty, the other side of the mountain."

The best part of learning to be alone and contented with your new self is all the surprises. For Mai, a woman of intense sexual desire, the first surprise was the ebbing of desire since she had entered menopause, for which she is grateful. "I couldn't relish my solitude right now if I had that old sexual urge pumping through my veins," she acknowledged. "I don't find it a loss, I find it a relief. It's allowing me to engage in the world in a different way than I ever have before."

Another surprise is that she is still attracted to men. A pile of bricks had sat in her yard for several months, like a burden of unremoved guilt, until she called up one of her male friends. She knew he was in the process of building an outdoor grill and thought he might want the bricks. He dashed right over with three of his friends. Mai watched these four bare-chested men bending and twisting and sweating in the sun and found herself turned on by their fierce male energy. She also found it easy to accept that she has not made a final either/or choice of sexual orientation.

"I'm not a radical person, but neither am I encumbered by what society or family might approve for me to do," she said. "The task of an artist, on one level, is to keep imagining how you can put things together. How can I put two clashing colors together on a canvas? Or how can I put these odd stones together to create something beautiful? And so you're re-creating your reality as you move along through time and space—you're always designing."

Chapter 17

A Nice Man to Visit, but I
Wouldn't Want to Live There

"*I* think my parents died of marriage."

That sassy remark may sound coldhearted at first, but this point of view on an older generation is growing among divorced and widowed women over 50. We know that the remarriage rate for women is not as high as it is for men. "It's assumed that's because women don't have enough available men; the guys can pick younger women, while women don't have as much choice," says Barbara Dafoe Whitehead, the co-director of the National Marriage Project. "That's an old-fashioned view. When a woman initiates a divorce in midlife, she asks herself, 'Why marry again when you can get a lot of what you enjoyed about marriage on your own?' This is especially true for women who have worked. They are more likely to prefer to remain single and enjoy romantic relationships. Also, if they have children, they're not eager to re-form another family and try to integrate children into it."

This attitude came through loud and clear in many of my interviews and e-mail responses. Truly seasoned women—and many seasoned men— are likely to prefer loving together and living apart, since both parties value their own space. Most women in this stage of life have adult children and one or more grandchildren, usually flung around the United States or the world and necessitating a lot of travel over holidays and vacations. It should come as no surprise that the new lover in the seasoned woman's life will not be all that crazy about traveling to Buffalo in December to spend Christmas with her grandkids. And he probably has his own to visit.

Moving in together may spoil a promising relationship, since the older we are, the more protective we are of our domain and lifestyle. What happens when he moves in with his "stuff" and is appalled at the pottery collection covering every surface in your house? A commonly repeated story is one like this: She collected antique dolls, he was a vintage sports car fanatic. When he moved in, it was hell. He went back to his place, and a few months later, they started seeing each other again but living apart, and it was sweeter than ever. She found it very romantic when he roared up in his vintage Porsche. And he was delighted when he could persuade this delicate lady to fold herself into the bucket seat and race around town with him.

Caroline, a 55-year-old northwestern woman, had to be eased into the delights of unmarried monogamy. She never thought she would find a man who could turn her on the way her husband had, but when his affairs had become too evident to ignore, she had to dissolve their marriage. When she was 50, she met a man who didn't want to marry again, had no interest in knowing her friends or family, and said he didn't believe in the idea of soulmates. He was clearly a workaholic and warned her that he was not boyfriend material. "But the pheromones were flowing, and he smelled and tasted awfully good to me," she said. "When we went to bed, it was as romantic as the fantasies I'd had as a teenager. I felt more sexual than I can ever remember. We don't talk about 'our relationship'; we don't use 'L-words'; and we never mention living together. My friends insist that I deserve someone who adores me, and they're amazed that I don't demand more from him. But with him I've had five years of sweetness, passion, and monogamy. Five years of being in the life and the bed of a man I adore. I have plenty of time for my friends, my children, my work, and being alone. Why would I wreck it by putting demands on a man for things he can't give?"

The obvious bonus of a longer-term visiting relationship is that it can retain some of the mystery and excitement of an affair. Since the main attraction of a new relationship for most of the single midlife women I've interviewed is romance, fun, companionship, and passionate sex, many wonder why they should put a damper on those attractions by falling into the "let's stay home and rent a movie," no makeup, no shower or perfume, heat up the leftovers, cozy couch potato habits that overtake most people who live together. Why put an end to "dating," that is, the fun of talking over plans for Friday night, getting your hair done, meeting at a restaurant, and wondering how the evening is going to end? Remember how Sandy's marriage sprang back to life after she and her estranged husband began "dating" again? People's living habits, almost indelibly ingrained by this age, don't have to grate on each other's nerves if they maintain separate spaces. It may be too late in life to train him to always use coasters, and maybe you don't want to give up your dog just because your lover is allergic to dog hair.

A Novel Prenuptial Agreement

Seasoned women and men are finding many different and creative ways to work out the balance between autonomy and dependence: How much time will they spend together, and what can they expect, and accept, that they will do separately?

One of the Passion Parties counselors I met in my travels saw her life make a 180-degree turn in the year she turned 50. Her story might sound like a romance novel, except that the ending is not "they lived together, happily ever after."

Nina Ward graduated from a Memphis high school in 1971 with no more promise than working at a Burger King. For most of her First Adulthood, she was a single mom who shifted between crummy $10-an-hour jobs and being on food stamps, always one step ahead of the repo man. That all changed when she moved to Fremont, California, and began working part-time for the company that was the precursor of Passion Parties. "I loved the money, I loved teaching and helping other women, giving them permission to enjoy their sexuality," Nina recalls. "It gave me a lot of self-esteem and confidence." After two years of giving parties, she quit her other jobs and threw herself into developing her business, only now and then remembering to date. In 1999, she won a silver star in the company's sales contest. She celebrated by dying her hair red and jazzing it up with a faux ponytail and tendrils. Her son was graduating from high school, her mother had just died, and she'd been single for fifteen years.

"So here I was, just fifty, no longer really a mother, a daughter, or a wife," says Nina. "I wanted to find out who Nina was, all by herself, without any label." By committing to dating over the Internet, Nina put herself into play. But she told her friends that she had no interest in getting married again. She was thoroughly enjoying cruising this new territory, when she was suddenly thrown into reverse.

The slow, sexy drawl of the surprise caller from Memphis was instantly recognizable to Nina. This was not one of her e-mail flirtations. This was Frank, her first love, the boy who had deflowered her when she was 16 and dated her until they were 19, when they suffered the adolescent torture of a first breakup.

There was silence on the line for a full minute before Frank blurted out his first full sentence. "In case anything happens to either one of us, I just want to apologize for everything that happened between us," he said. "It was all my fault." If there were ever a surefire way into a woman's heart, it's for a man to take all the blame. Frank sounded just as love-struck over her as he had when they were teenagers.

Nina's blood was racing, but her first words to him were "I don't know if you can handle me now, Frank. I'm a very independent woman."

This was May. She told him she probably couldn't make it to Memphis until October, but she held out for only two months. "When we first met again, it was instant hugging and kissing and crying, and we knew the attraction was still there." Nina flushes even in describing the meeting. "But we didn't know each other real well. So we went away for the weekend to a little bitty town in Arkansas, where the only room available was the honeymoon suite at the Best Western." Frank looked the same as he had in high school, but he had built a successful electrical contracting business. Nina, afflicted with the self-hating body image carried by so many women, apologized for the changes in her body: "I know I was thin and beautiful in high school, and I'm not anymore." Then she spoke from the new source of her self-esteem: "But I came from nothing, and now I'm making about $10,000 a month."

Frank was pleasantly shocked. He watched while Nina filled the

Jacuzzi with bubbles. She made him close his eyes before she would un- dress and join him. "Nina, I don't care about the changes in your body," Frank kept repeating. "I love you. I still think you're beautiful. I like that you're independent. That's good. And I make pretty good money now, too."

The prenuptial agreement was Nina's idea. "Which was huge for me," Nina says with a rolling laugh. "I never thought I'd be in a position where I would have reason to ask for a prenuptial agreement." The wed- ding took place in Tennessee ten months after their reunion. Since this would surely be her last wedding, Nina indulged in a full-length ivory gown, trimmed in beads and crystals, with a satin border. And being of an age to have a large number of close friends, she was attended by eight bridesmaids. But the most moving moment for Nina was when her son walked her down the aisle.

In the middle of the ceremony, Nina's minister instructed the couple, "Don't try to change one another."

Nina had no intention of hijacking Frank's life in Tennessee. She was also clear that she wasn't ready to leave behind the booming business she had built, the many friends who have become her support network, and being close to a son about to enter a state university—all in California. "I've always been with men who are very controlling and want to tell me what to do," says Nina. "They always say, 'I just want to protect you,' which really means they want to control you. I'm scared of losing myself in that cocoon." What's more, cultural attitudes toward a strong-willed, self-made businesswoman are still mixed in Tennessee at best, while in California Nina is roundly admired and acts as a mentor to younger women who, like her, began with nothing. No matter how much she loved Frank, giving all that up would inevitably lead to resentment.

Her solution is to commute between California and Tennessee, spend- ing two weeks of each month with Frank. She thinks she will probably keep it up for the next three or four years, until her son is out of college. By then, she and her husband may both be in a position to retire.

"Frank understands," Nina says, proud of their compromise. "We think it's going to keep our relationship hot! And I know it's going to help me ease into this marriage thing."

A Novel Postnuptial Agreement

Here is another creative way one married couple is managing to maintain their commitment to loving, honoring, and nurturing each other, but without living their daily lives together.

Mirjana is now in her serene sixties, softly pretty, with spiky black hair that lends a spark of youthful vehemence to the otherwise elegant colors and textures she wears. Her husband is fourteen years younger. When they married twenty-five years ago, she was a 40-year-old internationalist who was more than game to join in a gypsy life with her fiery Greek entrepreneurial partner and roam the world starting up small businesses. But the gap in their ages became much more glaring as they got older. Her husband is only now beginning to thrash around against "the little death" of his First Adulthood.

"He's approaching fifty—he may be having a midlife crisis, but that doesn't mean my life has to come to a screeching halt," Mirjana told me evenly. "We've had a lifestyle that I couldn't see myself continuing as I get older. Being fourteen years younger, he's still very high-energy and adventuresome. We've had businesses all over the world, and we still have several businesses together. But I'm not ready to pick up and run around the world anymore. I have two wonderful children from a previous marriage, and I'm a grandmother. As Grandma, you get another chance to do the pampering bit of mothering. At this stage of my life, I'm now more rooted in wanting to be around where my family is."

Mirjana's solution was to write a postnuptial agreement when the couple separated two years ago. "It's a permission, metaphorically, for him and for me to fly solo. It's about who I am as a person and what I love about him—and continue to love. And what I respect and honor in what we have achieved together. It's a promise that we will continue to love, nurture, and support each other until the day we die." She took care to render it with calligraphy to look like a diploma and framed it. Her husband told her he was very moved.

To her delight, they not only remain intimate, they make love almost as regularly as before their separation—and often with more passion. "Nothing has changed except that we don't live together," she says. "We're still married, but we both have the freedom to date. I don't really date. But if I do, I would want someone who can see beyond my aging. Yes, I am aging, but that's not who I am—my age. I don't get up in the morning and decide what I'm going to wear, I get up in the morning and dress to express my spirit."

It never occurred to Mirjana that she would start a new business of her own at 63. Using her psychology background, she has carved out a niche in the red-hot real estate market by "staging" people's homes for sale and helping families make the transition from leaving one home to furnishing the next. After only a year, she is wildly overbooked and loving every minute.

Mirjana says she used to be a classical victim: "I swear, if you woke me up in the middle of the night, I would say, 'Why me? Why did you do this to me?' " She produces fake sobs. "But now I believe that if you shook me awake in the middle of the night, I'd say, 'Hi, what do you want?' I've learned acceptance."

Part IV

The Boldness to Dream

*E*veryone knows of Julia Child, but did you know that she didn't go to cooking school until she was 36? And then it was a lark to amuse herself while she followed her husband to Paris after World War II. She tried out her first cooking show on TV only at the age of 51. The Julia Child who became the first celebrity chef, changing the way Americans think about food, was reborn as a new self in her Second Adulthood. Everything she was known for—a dozen cookbooks and an immensely successful TV show—she did after turning 50. Subsequently, she collected many honorary degrees in America and France and ultimately was awarded the highest honor in public television at the age of 87.

Women so often put off a half-formed dream in their First Adulthood. To revive that dream after 50 can infuse greater excitement than ever into life. So don't be discouraged if you have waited until now to become that person you always wanted to be.

Remember Julia Child.

Most of us reach midlife not knowing exactly what it is we want to do with the rest of our lives. A variety of techniques can help us home in on our hidden desires. Ask yourself, what has surprised you lately? If the answer is "Nothing," it's time to put yourself into an unfamiliar situation. Being in a new situation, especially one that holds a little danger— even the danger of embarrassment—stimulates the brain and opens up new and imaginative connections.

Think of Christo's gates, those furls of orange fabric with which the artist transformed New York's Central Park. Even the most familiar environment can be transformed into something wonderfully different, fresh, startling—we see it as if for the first time. When I took a walk through the gates on a snowy day, although I set out on my usual path, I became disoriented by looking up at the orange curtains billowing against the still, gray sky. They beckoned me in new directions, waved me on, and when I looked down again, I had lost my bearings. Delicious! I found myself on a path I had never known existed, which eventually took me around the back of the boating lake and rewarded me with a view completely new. This is exactly the effect that theater artists try to create. No matter how many times you may have seen *Carmen,* or *Carousel,* it is entirely new when you see a production by an innovative director such as Sir Peter Hall or Nicholas Hytner.

Try this exercise the next time you forget where you left your keys or your glasses: instead of rushing around the house in a frenzy, so that the blood vessels in your brain constrict and offer less oxygen to your thinking center, try retreating into a dark, quiet corner and meditating for five minutes—on any affirmation that isn't about keys or glasses. The answer might "come to you." The same process—in a much more elongated form, of course—is the most useful way I know to tap into your own unconscious wishes and allow your imagination to pick up on a passion that is just right for you: allow yourself ten minutes each day to sit in quiet and concentrate on what you want out of your Second Adulthood.

Here is a more sobering exercise: Imagine that you go to your doctor, you're told that you have a fatal disease, and you have only three months to live—but you'll be healthy until then. Ask yourself, if you had only three months to live, would you live them the way you did the last three? If the answer is "Definitely not," this is the time to change your focus; time to become shamelessly curious.

One of the greatest rewards of the previous phase—learning how to be alone with your new self—is likely to be the formation of outlines of a new dream. Inspiration is the first step, and not one that can be hurried; it might take months or even a year or two. Play with it. Don't just color inside the lines. Consider finding a coach.

We're old enough now to be mentors to younger aspirants, but no matter how old or young we are, we all need someone neutral to talk to. It might be a senior person in the field to which you aspire. It could be an acupuncturist or yoga teacher who is also eager to learn from working with you. It might be a friend ten or fifteen years your senior or a former professor whose zest for life is inspiring—just by periodically taking her or him out to lunch you will gain some life coaching. That was the idea behind the longtime best seller *Tuesdays with Morrie* by Mitch Albom. A life coach can teach you skills, help you over the humiliation of being a beginner again, build your confidence, and celebrate with you as you master your passion.

Once a year I try to spend a week at Rancho La Puerta, the health ranch in Mexico where the fitness revolution began back in 1940 (and where I learned strip dancing, as described in Chapter 15). When I'm there, I always meet women older than me who inspire me to go the distance. On an earlier stay I marveled at a compact, silvery-haired, 70-year-old woman from Indianapolis who passed me on the extended mountain hike, planting her hiking poles with jaunty determination as she moved in fluid full-body motion up the rocky path. The same woman turned up again in the Pilates class, and again in circuit training, and again in yoga. Finally, I caught up with her when she took a few minutes to read by the pool. Her name is Thelma Trudgen.

"What's your secret, Thelma?"

Her life coach was her mother, who had buried three husbands and was still going strong. "Mom's very competitive," she said. "That's what keeps her going, she wants to win at everything." Thelma told me a story to illustrate: "Mom was having a bridge party at her home in Gainesville, Florida, when a tornado came along. I saw it on TV and called her, very worried, but I couldn't get through by phone until that evening. She said, 'Oh, the tornado was terrible.' I said, 'Mom, tell me, what happened?' She said, 'Well, I was having a bridge party, and a tree fell right through the roof of our new house.' I said, 'What did you do?' She said, 'Well, the lights all went out, so we moved our tables closer to the window so we could see the cards!' I said, 'Mom, I'm going to go through life like that. Just keep moving.' "

Thelma took that insight literally. Her passion was hiking, but not just trudging the same old well-worn paths; she was walking the Appalachian Trail, state by state. Each year she and a hiking group of four women take a week to walk across the top of another state." We stay in nice bed-and-breakfasts," she admitted. "We like our glass of wine and a comfy bed." Thelma has crossed the mountains of Georgia, North Carolina, Tennessee, and Virginia, and was excited about hiking to the top of

Mount Katahdin in Maine the next autumn. Whenever I feel stuck, I picture Thelma—all five feet five of her—swinging her poles and walking up and down the world.

Sharing the Dream

One of the greatest potentials of a passionate life is to share the pursuit of a dream with your partner, especially at the empty-nest stage, when maximum freedom is combined with maximum capacities. You'll probably find that you both want a new meaning in life. It's not going to be raising children anymore, and it may not even be running another business. You've earned the right to a dream that isn't expected to pay the bills or appeal to the children. People who find a new dream or passion stay vital much longer than those who don't.

Of the happily married midlife couples studied by Dr. Judith Wallerstein, all found a new dream. Sometimes it's one they shared, but in other cases, each of them found a new direction. For your marriage to thrive, attention must be paid to your dream's impact on your partner, because dreams have unintended consequences. If there's no benefit to both from the partner's new dream, the inevitable by-product is resentment. Say he wants to go off to the African bush to do tropical medicine pro bono; where does that leave her, if she's thrilled about becoming head nurse at the local children's hospital and is devoted to her grandchildren?

In one of Wallerstein's couples, the woman became very involved in making art and her husband became deeply committed to fostering a venue for contemporary musical study and performance. They then had to renegotiate their household and their everyday way of life. They built a dual-use studio so she could paint and he could audition musicians. Their back-to-back dreams enhanced each other's creative pleasure. It may be that the best resolution for you is a dream that includes your husband. We'll read about a couple who worried about working together but found that blending their talents and passions actually enriched their marriage.

*   *   *

Sometimes our new dreams are born of disaster. Dr. Linda Hawes Clever confesses to having a congenital physician's personality. She is cautious, bordering on the obsessive, and tries to do everything to perfection. But, as she learned the hard way, "Life's trajectory can suddenly change." All the wheels began to come off in her fifty-eighth year: her mother died, her house was burglarized, she lost her "secure" hospital position and an editorship because of budget cuts, and within the same eighteen months her father died and her husband was diagnosed with prostate cancer. She might have gone down if not for her good friends, including John Gardner, the founder of Common Cause and a Stanford colleague. Linda asked Gardner to help her create a nonprofit organization to guide professionals to self-renewal before they burn out, or drop out of the medical field altogether.

"I surely looked like a candidate for self-renewal myself," says Linda. "This was a perfect opportunity to put theory into practice. With or without a catastrophe, how can people be stimulated to redream, refresh, and renew?"

The organization is called Renew. Dr. Clever holds workshops and seminars in San Francisco and across the country for doctors and nurses, teachers, leaders, and other hardworking, socially committed people, guiding them in how to anticipate the need to shift focus or how to find inspiration in adversity. Even more rewarding, she finds, are the informal conversation groups that get together in hospitals, clinics, or churches, where participants meet with a convener who offers life coaching and they all cheer one another along in a safe, collegial, fun environment.

When Renew offers a retreat, it isn't called a retreat; it's called an advance.

Chapter 18

Surviving *His* Midlife Crisis

*W*hat if the dream you have been carefully dribbling down the field toward your goal, like a soccer ball, is suddenly kicked out from under you by your mate's midlife crisis? A collision of new goals between a husband and wife as they kick off into the second half of the game of life, against the pressure of a faster-running clock, is a very common obstacle in the dream phase.

A common story in idyllic communities such as Santa Fe, which attract couples trying out a second act, often involves one partner dragging a mate behind him or her. After six months or a year, they often split up. People who want high-paying jobs or status seldom find them in small ponds. "You don't come to Santa Fe to make it," goes the local adage. "You make it and *then* come to Santa Fe."

One September morning in Santa Fe, my friend Marilyn Mason, a visionary writer and lecturer in her seventies who leads walking safaris in Africa and Tibet, collected a group of ten single seasoned women who were willing to talk about their experiences with love, sex, divorce, widowhood, living alone, and what came afterward. The women were candid from the start, and their candor was infectious. Some of their stories appear in other chapters, but here we will focus on the specific subject of surviving a mate's midlife crisis.

◆   ◆   ◆

Our hostess, Natalie Fitz-Gerald, greets our women's group rather formally, robed in a vivid ruby jacket with ropes of African beads spilling down the front and a cascade of multicolored hair falling to her shoulders. Standing still as a portrait, she is framed by the soaring openness of her two-story adobe living room with its massive freestanding stone fireplace and shelves full of African art. Natalie was born and raised in South Africa and became one of the first women to hold a seat on the Johannesburg Stock Exchange. She is elegant and cosmopolitan, with a velvety voice and an unerring artistic eye. But on closer look, something is wrong. A deep vertical furrow divides her brows. Her light blue eyes are lined in black and fringed a little too thickly with mascara, as if to screen the sadness in her heavily lidded eyes. Her jacket and loose black trousers disguise what looks like a body bloated with some extreme emotional overflow.

"I'm fifty-four, just going into menopause, and I'm dying!" She fans herself furiously. "I can't even imagine getting undressed in front of someone," she confides as we gather in the sun-splashed breakfast room, where she has organized a lavish meal for us. She is obviously a naturally gregarious person who loves the role of hostess and networker and has organized her large kitchen to produce buffets for big groups.

"My man dragged me here," Natalie explains. "He was having his midlife crisis, and he told me, 'Nothing lasts more than thirty years.' " She thought he meant only that he wanted to escape his first career as a highflier on Wall Street, get into sandals, and find somewhere other than New York City where he could live a quality life. She didn't guess that what he had in mind was discarding her. Natalie had given up her own career in finance to play the hostess–social director–cultural muse to the Great Man; her choice was to stick by him or retain her lively life in New York City. She chose him.

In Santa Fe, she threw herself into nonprofit efforts to promote women in the arts, joined a museum board, and shamelessly fund-raised for many organizations. She also established an annual New Year's Eve party for more than a hundred people in Santa Fe that became a coveted invitation. But there was one yearning that wouldn't be stilled: she had always wanted to create a gallery to display the dazzling array of arts and crafts from her native South Africa.

When she told her husband about the gallery idea, he was very dismissive. "You'd be no good at it," he said. It was less the lack of financial support than the contempt in his voice that deflated her dream. She put the idea on hold.

In her last-ditch desperation to hold on to the marriage, Natalie's gregarious spirit was suffocated. Her personality became distorted. Her usually robust self-confidence shrank even as her body blew up. And once her husband left, living alone in a big house geared to a robust social life was rather haunting. Nevertheless, once the path to divorce appeared inevitable, Natalie took a huge step toward consolidating her own identity: she became an American citizen.

"It was one of the proudest days of my life."

She had grown up in South Africa during apartheid. As a politically active college student, she had learned, firsthand, what it's like to fear the powers of a police state to whisk away anyone for speaking out and to hold him or her under detention without trial and with no recourse to the judicial system. One of her proudest acts as a new American and an independent woman was to allow herself to campaign for Kerry–Edwards. She made speeches and gave radio interviews. Hearing herself speak out about her core beliefs seemed to flip the switch, and she began to feel again like an independently thinking person, in touch with her African roots. Before her divorce settlement was finalized, she leased space for her gallery and made a buying trip to Africa. Within a week she had found enough unique rugs, pillows, pottery, and other artifacts to launch the dream of her Second Adulthood. And once she opened her doors, the patrons came, and appreciated, and purchased.

Natalie's dream gallery was barely a year old when she welcomed our group to her home. She admitted then that she was still reeling from the shock of divorce and not yet ready to try dating. But she assures us, "I am an enthusiastic survivor."

Six months later I interviewed Natalie again, this time catching up with her at her gallery, called Casa Nova. She was holding court in her office, where people drop by to discuss art or one of the many social projects they share with Natalie, or just to admire her latest love—a black-and-white pouf of a Pomeranian puppy curled in a doggie bed at her feet. Natalie's own demeanor was very different. Gone was the furrow between her brows. She was thinner. Radiant. Theatrically costumed in a saffron silk shirt with the collar flipped up and a handmade vest of flaming orange and turquoise—woven, she told us proudly, by women of Afghanistan. And no longer enduring hot flashes.

Shortly after our group meeting at her home, Natalie had told friends she was ready to date. Actually, she was feeling tremendous trepidation: "How do you start all over again? Is it back to the old style of dating?" She answered herself: "Of course not, because now we're all mature people. We've all been through the same kind of history, so there's a lot of common ground. The best way to handle it all is by joking. And by now I don't care. I feel that if someone is interested in me, they're interested in me because of who I am."

She even tried going on Match.com. She had a gazillon "winks" from men intrigued by her profile and went out with two men who turned out to be delightful. The boost to her self-confidence was enough to encourage her to throw the annual New Year's Eve party in 2004—by herself. It was, in a sense, her coming-out party.

The guest list was as eclectic as a grand buffet. They were nuclear physicists she has gotten to know at Los Alamos, rabbis and healers, dentists and doctors; judges and lawyers and mediation and arbitration experts she knows from her nonprofit work; opera people, chamber music people, theater people, and of course a heavy contingent of artists and designers. Her recipe is to mix male and female, toss with straight and gay, and add flavors from outside Santa Fe—friends with second homes here flew in from New York, even one friend from South Africa. She welcomed other people's holiday houseguests. The party was called "Flash and Glow," and the atmosphere was electric, partly because Natalie had found, online, rings that blink and leis and hair braids that flash, and as each guest came in he or she was adorned, until the whole house was lit up as if by fireflies in June.

The party swelled to 180 people, spilling over into every room. Truth be told, Natalie had been a little nervous about hosting such a large party on her own, but at the height of the festivities it hit her that none of the people she had pulled together seemed concerned about the absense of her husband. She might have met some of them with him or through him, but she had gone on to form independent relationships with them. She draws such a wide range of friends because she meets many people and quickly connects with them through her shameless curiosity. Her passion for intellectual pursuit is contagious. "I do a lot of reading, in all areas," she says. "And by mixing with these people, I learn. I pick up enough to have an intelligent conversation. I think that with a little bit of intuition and sensitivity, and some knowledge, you can hold your own with just about anyone."

It was an extraordinary evening. The next day she was deluged with phone calls from guests whose ubiquitous comment was "I can't believe what a great time I had—I met so many interesting people." Natalie, too, she told me with a wicked wink, had been introduced to a very special man. But she is not eager to hurry through this period of learning to live alone: "I'm enjoying dating because I am being so selective, and I'm not desperate."

Now that Natalie has survived her husband's midlife crisis and is moving through the Romantic Renaissance, her imagination is leaping ahead on a project that could be both commercially exciting and soul-satisfying: With the help of her contacts in the Third World, she is identifying rural cooperatives that are the result of poverty alleviation programs. She wants to help them market their products in the Western world. "I'll go over and work with them on design ideas and then come back to merchandise their products. We'll have Native American weavers go to South Africa and South African weavers come here . . ."

She can't stop talking about her dreams. It's the sound of a woman who has come far enough along the arc to have the boldness to dream big.

Chapter 19

Cashing In on the Sexual Diamond

A massive shift takes place across gender lines as we grow older. In *New Passages,* I described the geometry of this shift as "The Sexual Diamond" (see diagram). That is my way of visualizing the plasticity of gender characteristics over the course of our lifetimes.

Males and females are very much alike for the first ten years of life. We become radically differentiated at puberty and move to the farthest reaches of our oppositeness in our late thirties and early forties—the most distant poles of the Sexual Diamond. As we move into our fifties and beyond, both women and men take on many characteristics of their gender opposite, each becoming something of what the other used to be.

Anthropological studies, as well as empirical observation, tell us that men after 50 start to show greater interest in nurturing and being nurtured, in expressing themselves creatively or altruistically, and becoming more aware and appreciative of their surroundings. They remain identified with being male, but their need to prove themselves through sexual and aggressive conquest diminishes. They become more sentimental and emotionally vulnerable. Women, across cultures, age psychologically in the reverse direction, becoming more aggressive, managerial, and political. While they remain identified with being female, their focus is no longer diffused by caring for young children or the conflict between seduction and career achievement. Their tenderness and nurturing qualities become more broadly directed.

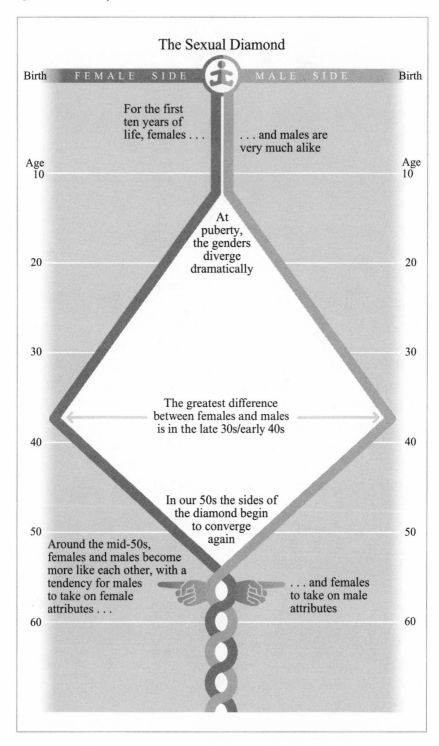

The Sexual Diamond

Birth   FEMALE   SIDE   MALE   SIDE   Birth

For the first ten years of life, females . . .

. . . and males are very much alike

Age 10   Age 10

At puberty, the genders diverge dramatically

20   20

30   30

The greatest difference between females and males is in the late 30s/early 40s

40   40

In our 50s the sides of the diamond begin to converge again

50   50

Around the mid-50s, females and males become more like each other, with a tendency for males to take on female attributes . . .

. . . and females to take on male attributes

60   60

Around 50, however, men and women may run into a rather stark dy-synchrony in their passages. As men's careers reach their peak and start winding down, either by choice or involuntarily, women's aspirations, often postponed by familial responsibilities—as we've discussed—are likely to be revving up. One of the most dramatic changes in our social balance is the fact that so many women in their forties and fifties today are holding down good jobs. There is nothing unusual about a midlife woman entrepreneur applying for a bank loan to start a new business or a nonprofit, or to go to graduate school. Nor is it unusual today for a high-performing career woman to have babies or adopt, in her forties, and continue her career. These women are usually exhilarated about new possibilities in their Second Adulthood, while, in some cases, their hus-bands may be slowing down, topped off or simply bored and wanting more hands-on attention.

Couples should not be surprised by a switch of polarities in marriage. But rather than the sexes' simply trading roles in middle life, men and women are freer to express both the masculine and feminine sides of their personalities. We have the chance to reach a point of harmony—the upper point of the Sexual Diamond—where the tension of male-female differences relaxes at last.

Those women and men who have made previous passages with guile and grace, and accept that change is good, natural, and essential, can welcome the new equity in relationships now possible for the next thirty or forty years of our lives.

That's the beauty of a long and seasoned marriage: the evolution of "we." This is the stage when a couple can cash in on the Sexual Dia-mond. The reward for making it into midlife together is a true mutuality, where giving and receiving are equally pleasurable. It forms the core of middle and later life, as precious as good food, bodily closeness, emo-tional empathy, and uninhibited sex. Mutuality means that each of you is able to get inside your partner's skin to *feel* how he or she feels and in-stinctively know how best to respond.

The Sexual Diamond can be realized most easily in a mature cou-ple who enjoy working together in a business or on a project, cause, or major life endeavor. The worth of each one's contributions is affirmed from day to day. If a true complementarity is played out in the realm of work, it becomes more natural as the basis for compromise in the personal realm.

A Very Complementary Couple

Like many women of her generation, Elaine Petrocelli started out as a schoolteacher. A starry-eyed do-gooder in the late Sixties, Elaine secured a million-dollar grant for her nonprofit school to combat racism, only to discover that a high-level employee there was keeping two sets of books. Elaine turned for advice to an attorney she had just begun dating, Bill Petrocelli, who was on the school's board. When Bill had to shut down the school, it might have been the death knell of Elaine's idealism. Instead, Bill asked Elaine, "What are you passionate about?"

"Books," she said. "This may be a really dumb idea, but I've always wanted to be a bookseller."

Not only did he encourage her to follow her passion, they got married. Twenty-nine years later, Elaine is one of the swelling legions of small-business owners—the greatest proportion of whom are women. She is the long-standing proprietress of Book Passage in the hills of Marin County, where she employs a happy tribe of sixty men and women booksellers with whom she insists upon sharing credit.

Elaine never seems to stop smiling. She wasn't able to change the world, but she has done the next best thing. You see her passion when Elaine glides through her bookstore on little sandaled feet, her smoky green eyes darting right and left, not missing a trick, appraising everything from the point of view of the book buyer. Her silver hair frames her face in soft waves, everything very natural. Bill Petrocelli, tall and muscular, backs her up with a solid masculine presence. "Elaine is always three steps ahead of me," he says without a trace of tattered ego.

But that is not quite the truth. It was Bill who designed and oversaw the construction of a second building as their bookstore expanded. Book Passage has become much more than a store; it's a cultural center. Writers and readers are encouraged to meet and exchange ideas, which are then transmitted by Elaine to publishers: "*This* is what your readers really want."

Bill was formerly a tough attorney in San Francisco. He listened to

Elaine complain that the discounts publishers gave the chains were surely more generous than those given to a store like hers, so why would any sane person want to be an independent bookseller? Bill began to investigate. The couple became active in the Northern California Independent Booksellers Association and ended up participating in a fair trade lawsuit filed against two major publishers. Bill was the attorney. "We've managed to stop a few unfair practices," says Bill. "It's a constant battle. It's like the Hundred Years' War. But we have made it clear to publishers that they need us as much as we need them."

As Bill spent more and more time working in the bookstore, he noticed that everyone on the staff showed up there in a happy mood. "It was totally different than when I went to my law office and everyone showed up angry." He was hungering for a change in midlife; why not join his wife's business?

"I was scared he might come in and take over," Elaine admits, adding, with her ready laughter, "or maybe we would fight. If you have a disagreement with your spouse and you're in business, you're likely to fight in front of sixty employees. Bill had to make himself valuable." Her husband quickly proved himself useful by wielding spreadsheets and acting as the legal hammer behind Elaine's emollient public personality. "Now Bill is a seven-day-a-week guy," she says. "Sometimes I say to him, 'Go home!'" She giggles. "I don't think there are too many couples who work together and are happy about it. But for us, for me, it's better, because we're so involved. If I were married to someone who didn't share this passion of mine, there probably would be resentment. He'd say, 'She doesn't do anything all day except meet famous authors!'" As it is, Elaine reads a new book almost every night. "Bill and I read together," she clarifies. "It's something we enjoy doing together in the evening."

The Petrocellis are not only in the book business; they're in showbiz. Their store hosts between five hundred and seven hundred author events in a year. Elaine or Bill or their events coordinator is sworn to actually read the book before introducing the author, which explains why Book Passage is a favorite destination for authors on tour. That's probably why Simon & Schuster chose Book Passage out of dozens of other fine booksellers in the San Francisco Bay area to send Hillary Clinton to for the debut of her best seller *Living History*. They sold more than two thousand copies of Hillary's book the first day—all the copies they could get their hands on.

But to keep their marriage fresh, the Petrocellis had to find a refuge. They needed a time and place to imagine how to make their lives more meaningful and give back. On their fifteenth anniversary, Elaine persuaded Bill to buy a small house in Italy to which they could escape to dream. As they walked together beside the serene Lake Guarda in northern Italy, Bill asked Elaine if there were anything that she was missing in life.

"Teaching," she admitted. "This may be a really dumb idea, but what if we started a conference for travel writers?"

That was Bill's cue to get out the yellow pad and figure out how to make Elaine's vision work. Elaine made a cold call to the travel editor at the San Francisco *Examiner,* Donald George, who was so enthusiastic, he phoned the famous travel writer Jan Morris, who answered in her bathtub in Wales and agreed to come. The first conference was such a hit, it is now in its fourteenth year and has spawned hundreds—literally hundreds—of working, earning, professional travel writers.

Elaine's enthusiasm and graciousness have also made Book Passage a haven for serious authors. In the late Eighties, when Isabel Allende met her husband, he brought her to Book Passage to buy a book. "Elaine and I became friends," Allende told me, "and Book Passage became like my refuge. My husband had a tiny house at the time. His children were very small, and domestic life was chaotic. There was no place to be. So I started coming here to read, to research, to do all of my interviews in the coffee shop. This was my office. From '87 until '90."

Later, when Elaine was out for several months with a health problem, Allende returned the favor. "One morning I stumbled in to teach a class for the travel writers' conference," recalls Don George, "and did a double take at the tiny woman in an apron behind the café counter who made my latte. Aren't you—?"

Yes, it was the very same woman whose portrait hangs in the store above the "shrine" of her twelve books: Isabel Allende.

As Elaine has become more aggressive and managerial in her Second Adulthood, Bill has become more reflective and creative. His love now is writing the store's opinionated bimonthly newsletter, which is mailed to forty thousand people. Elaine is now in her mid-sixties and has fully integrated her first love—teaching—with her passion for bookselling. So magnetic is her enthusiasm for her vocation that her daughter has now joined the family business and her son participates as well. "I think that they feel they can do this because they have watched Bill and me work well together."

The Petrocellis now keep their store humming like a small college, fondly nicknamed BPU, Book Passage University. They also run four-day writing conferences, which have turned the store into a petri dish where the couple cultivate new writers and build lasting customer loyalty. "But these things didn't start as smart business ideas," Elaine demurs. They started, like most of this seasoned couple's inventions, with Elaine saying to Bill, "This is probably a dumb idea, but . . ."

The Petrocellis are more than just Bill and Elaine. As with any couple who have achieved the sexual diamond, the evolution of "we" leads to a much greater and stronger being, capable of achieving far more than they would on their own. Their growth as a couple is manifested in the growth of their company.

Chapter 20

Crossing the Sexual Border in Midlife

*K*aran comes bustling out of the kitchen where she has been happily preparing a buffet, licking fudge batter off her fingers and swinging her tumble of honey blond curls. She is a busty, broad-bottomed, exuberant woman, and as she welcomes me into the Triangle Inn she blurts out, "I lost my hair from medical treatment, and I couldn't wait to grow it back. My partner liked it short, but hey"—she tosses her mane proudly—"I can't be Barbie with short hair!"

Being a Barbie works perfectly for Karan. She's a self-proclaimed girly-girl, wearing her nails long and painted, constantly puttering around her Santa Fe inn, answering the phones, mothering the guests, and adding pretty touches to the place. Her "Ken" takes care of everything else—plumbing, carpentry, heavy lifting—which suits her just fine. The couple is preparing to host a group interview for my benefit, complete with an open mesquite-fire hearth and margaritas. When the phone rings, Karan is bent over the oven, pulling out homemade brownies. "Ken" picks up the call and says, "You'll need to wait to talk to Karan. She takes care of the social stuff."

Karan relishes her traditional female role in what she calls her "Fifties-style marriage," and not just because it allows her to revel in all aspects of femininity. "We've been together for fifteen years, and of course there are ups and downs. But we're very serious about our relationship. We're committed to staying together. Infidelity is forbidden. So even after the worst fights, when we both go off to sulk, we tell ourselves, 'Well, I'm in a Fifties-style marriage. I guess I've gotta stay.' "

It would be easy to picture Karan on a black-and-white Fifties TV screen, happily vacuuming in an apron and pumps, except for two glaring inconsistencies: At the age of 50, she's been divorced twice. And her "Ken" is no muscle-bound man but Sarah—a finely boned woman of 42.

Sarah, the granddaughter of a midwestern governor, comes from a moneyed family. "I was raised to go to Wellesley, excel academically, and marry a Harvard or MIT man," Sarah tells me. "But I always knew who I was, and it was hard to reconcile the family dream with being a lesbian." Sarah didn't want to miss out on having a child, but in her era, that seemed impossible without a male mate. So instead of focusing on her love life, she devoted herself to her career and soon rose to a high management position at a Washington, D.C., firm.

It was in D.C., in her thirties, that she met and fell in love with Karan, an older woman from a lower-middle-class background who had started out working as a secretary and, by virtue of grit and talent, become an assistant development director who organized fund-raisers for up to five hundred people. In their first three years together, the two women worked out most of their demons and moved into a dream house together on Capitol Hill. "I had a secure job with a top firm," Sarah says. "I was in a top management position with great money, great benefits, five weeks' vacation—and I was miserable."

"We never saw each other," Karan explains. "We were both working eighty hours a week and completely stressed out. We wanted to change our lives from running the big-city rat race and instead work on our relationship, rather than just occupying the same house."

They were soon presented with one of those life accidents that turns out to open a new door. When Karan and Sarah came out publicly as a couple, Karan was fired, despite six years of glowing reports. They decided to use the opportunity to change their lifestyle. Karan's mother, who lived in Santa Fe, was getting older and needed more care. Karan considered moving her mother to the East Coast, but she knew she'd be miserable. So instead, Sarah and Karan went out to Santa Fe to look at real estate.

"We tumbled down a road and saw this place—and here we are, eleven years later," says Karan. "This place" was a charming, though at the time ramshackle, assortment of pueblo-style *casitas* at the base of the Santa Fe foothills. Cottonwood trees dotted the landscape. Buying it, and making the massive renovations necessary to turn it into a functioning inn, took all of their resources and represented as great a commitment as most married couples make. "This is not a moneymaking experience," says Karan. "Owning a bed-and-breakfast is seriously downwardly mobile, but—"

Sarah jumps in: "In Washington, we had money but no time to enjoy it. Now we have lots of time and no money."

"But," Karan interrupts, "Sarah has a nice extended family that has done well, and they like to fly us to foreign countries and house us and feed us. And they come and stay at the inn. Sarah's sister got married here."

Becoming innkeepers was only a goal at first, but, infused with their love for each other and the sense of liberation they felt, it snowballed into a larger dream—to provide a holiday escape for other women like themselves. Most of the women who stay at the inn are in couples relationships. "We love the interaction with the lesbian community," says Karan. "Recently, we had an obvious transsexual as a guest. No other place in town would have taken her. We love being able to provide a shelter for people like that."

With the Greatest of Ease

Although Karan and Sarah's is not a conventional union, their relationship does fit Dr. Judith Wallerstein's thesis of what makes a good marriage. They anticipated the need to change their lives and did so in their thirties. They took a bold (and financially perilous) risk to make a new dream a living reality. And their sexual intimacy continues to replenish their emotional bond.

It was intriguing that of the lesbian couples they gathered together for our group interview, all but Sarah had previously identified themselves as heterosexual. They had been married to men and valued that experience, expressing no bitterness. And most had had children. They themselves were surprised by the ease with which they had made the internal transition from being straight to finding love with another woman. All of them had done so sometime between their mid-thirties and fifties. They all seem to have formed a valid relationship with another woman and to be leading unapologetic, successful, even ordinary lives.

I wondered if this trend—previously heterosexual women sliding easily into a lesbian lifestyle at midlife—was unique to this quirky, artistic Santa Fe group, or if it was a larger and unpublicized trend. I looked into it and was surprised to find that research on this phenomenon was practically nonexistent. The only study I could find was a 2004 thesis by Victoria University doctoral candidate Kristin Henry entitled "Dancing Across Borders: Women Who Become Lesbians in Mid-Life." The study's most startling finding was that many of the twenty-eight women interviewed insisted that they could not have crossed the sexual border until they had first crossed the territory from youth into middle age. Midlife allows a woman to stop living solely by societal norms and instead shape her lifestyle into something that is more in line with *her* ideals.

The author was surprised by the ease of this midlife switch: "I wanted the women who participated in the research to tell me, 'Yes, it is very difficult sometimes.' Instead, I discovered that lots of women had found the transition so easy, and so rewarding, that they had never looked back." Their reasons for becoming lesbians had nothing to do with the availability of men—in fact, men had had little to do with the decision at all.

Like the women in my Triangle Inn group interview, most of the twenty-eight women who participated in Ms. Henry's thesis study had felt affection, in varying degrees, for their previous male partners. Many had enjoyed heterosexual sex and some believed they still could under the right circumstances. Some acknowledged that they had been relatively happy wives. Most of the twenty-eight were mothers, and those who were tended to feel that motherhood was at least as much of a defining factor in their identity as their sexuality, if not more.

*   *   *

Six months after Karan and Sarah hosted the group interview at their Triangle Inn, we met at the Village Market, a funky breakfast café in the New Mexico village of Tesuque on the outskirts of Santa Fe. They couldn't wait to tell me about the reunion with Sarah's Wellesley dorm mates, the Pom 13, who had lived together in the Pomeroy Hall dorm. The other twelve women had fulfilled the expectations of their tribe, marrying and remaining married to their male Ivy League counterparts. Sarah had invited them all out to celebrate with her and Karan.

"We had much more in common, from living with the same person for so many years, than the difference in our sexual leanings," says Sarah. Karan chimes in, "We are more married than any heterosexual couple. There's no mine and hers with us. It's all ours."

The closeness and communication they share are now allowing Karan and Sarah, at 50 and 42, to pursue a fresh dream: they are going to try to have a child. They've begun researching the various options that technology now allows lesbian couples. And they've decided that Sarah will carry the baby. She's younger and doesn't have the genetic baggage of medical conditions that Karan does. Despite the fact that their new dream goes against the traditional roles they have adopted until now, they're thrilled with this exciting new prospect.

"One of the reasons I had such a hard time coming out was because I really wanted children," Sarah repeats. Between trips to the doctor's office, Sarah is working on turning one of the *casitas* into a three-room nursery suite. "So there *will* be children," she declares. "If you build a nursery, they will come."

Part V

Soul Seeking

*A*s we grow older, we want to grow wiser. In my interviews, people who were thrilled to be swept up in a Romantic Renaissance often described a dramatic new transition as they moved into their late fifties or sixties. A hunger wells up for another dimension of experience—a greater depth of meaning and value in the activities of everyday life. A spiritual expansion.

We become more sensitive to our place in the larger scheme of things. We are drawn to flashes of the sacred in people, places, and art that feed the soul. Some people are moved to make a spiritual quest. Others are called back to the religious tradition in which they were raised, or they intensify their family rituals. Still others do not relate this hunger to any religious belief or church attendance, but feel the need to stretch beyond self and even relationships, toward a deeper appreciation of a collective intelligence working in the universe: a soul connection.

The soul is not an easy concept to define. I think of it as the essence. We all have an essence; it was there when we were born, before all the experiences by which we are shaped and that form the edifice of our personality and defenses. We rarely see that essence in ourselves or recognize it in others, until life trips us up. Soul thrusts up from below, through the cracks of our daily existence and when things fall apart. Inevitably, at some point in our fifties or sixties, most of us will face a crisis of great magnitude, such as when a serious illness strikes us or our partner, or one or the other is ruthlessly devalued in the workplace. Unpredictable life accidents such as these strip away the edifice of our well-defended lives. We are forced to look inside for the presence of soul in ourselves and to perceive the qualities of soul in others.

Seeking soul is not the same as seeking a cure. Seeing a professional to help solve a painful situation is very different from making room for the slow, quiet, subjective observance of your own soulfulness. In his thoughtful book *Care of the Soul,* the theologian and former Catholic monk Thomas Moore suggests, "The human soul is not meant to be understood. Rather, you might take a more relaxed position and reflect on the way your life has taken shape. . . . If you attend the soul closely enough, with an educated and steadfast imagination, changes take place without your being aware of them until they are all over and well in place."

In times of passage, the soul may lose itself. We feel intensely fallible, uncertain of the ground beneath us, of whether or not we really have an essence of our own. In times like these I try to find the way back by going deep into nature, walking in the woods, climbing hills, sitting on a rock above a crashing sea, until I sense some wild creature inside myself that responds to the ferocity of life. That creature feels like something deep in the core that would know how to survive when will is not enough.

Seeking a Soulmate

Most of us would love to have a soulmate to share our life. But the term "soulmate" is too often tossed around in a very superficial way, as if it were something to hope for from a blind date or a qualification for choosing your favorite hunk on *American Idol.*

"The search for a soulmate can sometimes trip people up," says Dr. Melanie Horn, a seasoned psychologist with a San Francisco practice full of high-expectation patients. "A lot of women come into my office and say, 'I have this really nice relationship, but I'm not sure he's my soulmate.' They may not recognize that the way you have a soulmate is by sharing your soul with another person over time. Sometimes it happens in the process of accepting differences. If you can let each other be, it can lead to understanding and real sharing."

Jane Fonda reveals in her autobiography that she has been searching for her own essence all her life. After years of bulimia and anorexia, three divorces, and becoming a Christian, Jane Fonda is 67 years old, lives alone, and has been celibate for the last couple of years. She told Larry King in a CNN interview, with breathless expectation, that she had recently visited a psychic, who had told her that "I'll meet my soul-mate in the next year."

We don't *meet* a soulmate. We *forge* a soulmate. We all long to be seen and loved in our essence. Yet most of us are guarded, especially if we have been battered by life and lost a love or two. It is when another person is able to connect with your essence, and you with his or hers, that a soulmate connection is forged. You have to be willing to risk that depth of attachment, which means surrendering some control, moving beyond ego-driven narcissism, exposing some of the holes in your soul, and inviting intimacy. That usually takes at least a few years of giving and receiving love, testing trust, and coming to believe that we are loved just for what we are. All the rest is background music.

◆　　　◆　　　◆

The middle and later years are the optimum time to connect on a deeper level with a soulmate—a person who recognizes and loves the seeker in you. Yeats called it the "pilgrim soul." It could be your husband, if he appreciates your evolving identity over and above your changing face and body. In fact, couples who have been together for a long time have a great opportunity to enrich and anchor their relationship in the course of weathering crises of the soul together. A couple that reaches that level of love—a connectedness of soul to soul—forges a container as solid as pure gold to hold their love and commitment as they move toward the passage to the Age of Unity.

Many of the single women I've interviewed, once they move into the late fifties, find their priorities changing significantly. Now they are more eager to find a true friend and partner in life, someone who will be interested in joining them in a larger cause, such as protecting the environment or mentoring at-risk children, or who is ready to look together for a place in the sun where they could eventually retire. The soulmate is often a rediscovered first love. It might be a formerly married friend or a person met almost anywhere who is on a parallel journey. Surprisingly often, it is found in a platonic relationship with someone who is a trusted and inspirational companion in seeking the soulful life.

Men, as they grow older, are especially prone to sex and death anxieties. They are constantly bombarded with ads for Viagra and the steroidal mania that turns thirty-something baseball players into freak Hall of Famers and teenage sons into testosterone dopers. All that hoopla cannot help but remind older men that they may have trouble competing in the contemporary athletic and sexual carnival, especially if they still think of sex as a competitive sport. Death anxieties are fueled by the suddenness of heart attacks felling their friends. At an even deeper level, men as they get older may be bedeviled by feeling a lack of meaning in their life. Men's depression is claiming increased attention from the National Institute of Mental Health. The highest suicide rates are found in men over age 65, ten times as many of whom kill themselves as do women.

A life crisis can be a gift at this stage, because it forces the individual to confront the givens of existence: aging, suffering, death, the necessity of loving and being loved, the need for one's life to add up to something. When any one of us begins wrestling with these eternal questions, we are seeking a spiritual framework whether we acknowledge it or not.

The psychotherapist Irvin Yalom, who writes about existential therapy, told me his view of psychotherapy is a venture in learning how to be intimate. He finds this approach particularly helpful in working with older executive men and CEOs, who are almost forced into isolation in the workplace. "They have no peers, they can't establish friendships with people who work under them, they keep fewer friends from the past than women do," he observed. "So when they feel vulnerable about aging or illness or winding down, they suffer an isolation from within. That can lead to a preoccupation with death, or suicide. Things they can't say to people who care about them, they can say when you get them into a safe situation like therapy. There can be great exhilaration in dropping the mask."

As more and more Europeans and Americans resist the strict dogma of the churches in which they were raised, there is more talk of spiritual quests and soul seeking. Many Christians I know combine a little bit of Jesus, a little bit of yoga, some private prayer, some social activism in the public square, and perhaps inspiration from the divine feminine. Feminist scholarship, the evocations in popular culture of a redeemed Mary Magdalene as Jesus' beloved, and reminders of the naked imposition of patriarchy by the medieval Church—as in *The Da Vinci Code,* by Dan Brown, and in *Goddesses in Older Women,* by Jean Shinoda Bolen—all combine to encourage women to sort out their own religious feelings and to redefine spirituality. Jewish feminists, missing their own reflections in the myriad of religious practices, are defining their own spirituality and rituals. The Jewish feminist organization Ma'yan has created a thirty-year tradition of feminine-focused seders, where as many as twenty thousand women have gathered across the country and overseas to sing, dance, and go through the ritualized retelling of the Jewish liberation story, emphasizing the woman's experience.

It's never too late to make a soul connection. We will hear the story of a widow and widower in their mid-sixties who met and married within a year; a decade later, they have become the closest of soulmates. But it's important to qualify their story so it doesn't read as a fairy tale. Both partners brought vital elements of character and experience to their late-life match. They are both blessed with a positive outlook and a fun-loving nature; both had been in charge of their own careers and achieved admirable success and public recognition; and perhaps most important of all, before death took their first partners, both of them had known happy marriages. They knew what it takes.

Chapter 21

"I'm Giving Up Younger Men"

"*I*'m sorry, I don't date anyone under forty-five anymore."

That is the new rule laid down by Bebe, the jazz singer and poster girl for dating after 50 whom I met in an Oakland restaurant, and describe at the beginning of this book. Only a seasoned woman could casually utter such a line to a bedazzled young man.

At 50, Bebe had left her emotionally immobilized husband and plunged into a long Romantic Renaissance, seven years of surfing the edges of relationships with men of all ages and stations in life. Her propensity was to go for much younger men, starting with her first encounter at church, when a handsome and hot young guy teased out the fact that she was separated and insisted they go out to lunch. That romance quickly swelled into six months of sexual bliss and romantic playfulness, but, as Bebe expected, it receded as carelessly as it had erupted.

She learned how to be alone when she had to comfort herself through a hysterectomy. It prepared her to take advantage of the dormant periods in between intense romances to rest, write in her journal, and replenish her spiritual connections. She also had more time to work on a new dream that could take her beyond her performing years.

Currently 57, Bebe has felt a major internal shift. With some reluctance, because she loved all her flings, she acknowledges that at this stage she is less interested in short-term romance and hungry for something much more soulful. "What I'm looking for at fifty-seven does not mesh with what a man of thirty-seven is thinking about—men in their thirties

and early forties are still climbing in a hurry to get to the top and thinking about getting their kids through high school," she tells me at one of
our follow-up interviews. We meet in a popular club in the Berkeley hills,
the Paragon, which on a Friday night draws a sophisticated crowd of
mostly black professionals of middling age who eat, drink, and table-
hop on an outdoor terrace overlooking San Francisco Bay.

Bebe is a brandy-skinned African-American woman who is utterly
fearless about flirting. Leading with an ample bosom under a zippered
pink sweater, she insinuates herself through the men and women standing three-deep around the bar, stopping for effusive greetings to casual
acquaintances, and a radar-eyed scan of potential romantic marks. Her
laugh is as intoxicating as the tropical-fruited drinks. Always the bold
one among her friends, Bebe has no hesitation about starting up a conversation. When she spots "her type" at a table—a lean man with a brain
bulge exposed by his close-shaven skull, a sly mustache, and sloe eyes—
she would ordinarily have no compunction about sashaying over and ad-
dressing him and his four male dinner companions.

Spooning out her thickest southern drawl: "Now really, don't you
men think you should integrate this table with at least one woman?"

Of course, they would eagerly invite her to join them and the banter
would begin. Except that tonight, Bebe is in a dormant phase. She doesn't
approach the table, because once you lay down your cards, she says, you
have to be ready to play out the hand. She's not ready tonight. Over the
winter she had two strong relationships going simultaneously, each of
which tapered off for different reasons. She is reorienting her priorities.
What she is looking for now is what most of us want as we feel the sun
setting a little sooner every day: a soulmate. In particular, Bebe is looking for a kindred spirit who could share her appetite for adventure and
travel, her dreams of social activism, and a second home in the sun where
eventually they could retire.

"He has to be a passionate person," she insists. "I don't mean necessarily sexually passionate, but passionate about life. He has to enjoy just
getting up in the morning and doing whatever he does." It isn't easy to fill
such an order among men over 50, she laments. "They worry about getting older, they worry about not being productive, they worry about not
having enough money, they worry about not looking good—they worry!

So they're not much fun. Maybe it's just what happens to men when they get past fifty, compared to what happens to women. I think we blossom after fifty. I think men get scared. They tend to think their world is ending."

"Can you restore the magic for those men?" I ask her.

"Uh-huh," Bebe replies glumly. "But I don't want that job. I had that job with my husband. I don't want to be responsible for somebody else's happiness. I want him to be able to be happy on his own." She flashes a dazzling smile. "But then be happier with me."

Some of Bebe's strongest attributes are initially appealing but eventually intimidating. "They love the fact that my brain works so fast, but it's also what they come to hate," she says with a laugh. "They say, 'You're always thinking!' " Being an entertainer, she has many social connections and finds herself comfortable in all kinds of situations, which can make her dates feel overshadowed.

Perhaps because she is so accomplished and confident, the men she dates sometimes inflate their history. She's become quite skilled at picking up clues to a fraud. The second time they have a conversation about his college years, she may get a "ping" when he mispronounces the name of his fraternity. "If I get too many pings, I start checking." More than once she has hired a private investigator to check out men who sounded too good to be true. Her instincts were usually correct.

"I've never gotten bitter, even when things haven't worked out with men I had hoped would remain in my life," says Bebe. That lack of bitterness is an important ingredient in her continuing appeal. Whether or not there is a man in her life, Bebe makes certain to refresh herself with new experiences and new people. This gives her an endless source of charisma. But at this stage in her pursuit of the passionate life, Bebe is not willing to take as many risks as in the past. She is wary of a man's health status. She is realistic about the fact that illness is likely to invade a midlife relationship and is more likely to strike the man than the woman. At dinner with a new man, she teases out as much as she can about his lifestyle and makes mental notes about his health profile. "By the second date, if I see he's having too many drinks, it's a ping—how many drinks does he have when he's home alone?"

What scares her the most about getting serious with an older man is that he might get sick and expect her to take care of him. "I don't feel I'm cut out for that role." She has never had children. Whatever maternal urges she has are well satisfied by being the Auntie Mame to her nephews, the children of a sibling who tragically died, and to the sons and daughters of close friends.

Here lies a paradox for the older single woman who is seeking a soulmate. Not only does commitment to an older man carry the risk of eventually becoming a caregiver, it is virtually a certainty that at some point one of you will take ill. What makes periods of illness bearable, when the normal routines and many of the pleasures of life are suspended, is the bond of souls. That depth of attachment is acquired through sharing the pain and pleasures of many years together. When love goes that deep, it embraces body and soul. The body is the canvas on which the soul paints the shapes and colors of a person's silhouette, skin tone, animation, or ennui, and displays its contentments and distempers in posture, pain, and the symptoms of disease.

It is hardly realistic for a woman to expect to feel the same bond with a "significant other" who has been in her life for only a year or two. And the older she is, the more likely a relationship will encompass periods of illness. But, as Bebe is discovering, there are other sources of nurturing and caring that do not depend on a sexual relationship.

Revealing Your Own Soul

Many people who find themselves without a soulmate at this stage of life are moved to make a greater effort to know their own soul. Some set off on a spiritual quest. Others seek revelation through psychotherapy. Bebe is aware that she must sustain herself on her own essence, since there is currently no partner to reflect it back to her. But there is also a divine presence in her life. "I'm not a churchgoer," she says. "But I'm a very spiritual person, and that's what sustains me through tough times. I think as you get older, your relationship grows stronger with whatever you consider the Great Being, whether you call it God, Yahweh, or Mohammad. You see it work in your life, you refine it, and you know how you tap into it. It's a quiet presence.

"When I don't have what I want, I make peace with what I have," she says philosophically. "You can lose so much energy worrying about what you don't have. That doesn't mean you have to stop dreaming or stop working on what you want, and it doesn't mean you won't have it the next time around."

This may be what Bebe's seasoned years will look like. Given her low tolerance for the risk of a committed relationship at this stage, she is finding a new category of companions, whom she calls "romantic friends." These are men, some straight, some gay, who enjoy going to the theater with her, having a nightcap, kissing hello and good-bye, and that's it. She is also building her network of women mates. The week before we talked, she had gone to Chicago for a weekend of theater and shopping, where she had "dates" with two of her male "romantic friends." On Sunday, Bebe and several of her girlfriends took her god-daughter to the elegant tearoom at the St. Regis Hotel for jasmine tea and scones, after a whirlwind shopping spree. Bebe laughed at hearing her godchild's impression of her life.

"Aunt Sugar," she said, "I like the way you and your girlfriends hang out. You guys look fabulous, you have younger boyfriends, you travel everywhere. I'm thinking I'm going to be like you when I get old."

"Old!" Bebe sputters with a deep laugh. "But she's seeing that a woman's life doesn't have to be either/or—either you're married to a man you're going to be with forever, or you're going to be an old maid sitting around the fire alone. I'm glad that the daughters of my generation see us living in our fifties in a very different way. They will begin to see that their future, too, can take different paths."

Chapter 22

Surprise Soulmates

soulmate can be hardest to find when you're looking for one. It seems to happen serendipitously—after you decide that you are perfectly content living independently. This paradoxical truth was born out for two midwestern women, Kalli and Elizabeth, whose pursuits of the passionate life took them in opposite directions.

The two Chicago women had become fast friends over their shared interest in Greek antiquities, around which each of them had framed successful careers. Both women had married men of quality, and from time to time they had envied each other. Neither would have predicted that the other's seamless life would suddenly fall apart.

Kalli is a pretty woman with large dark eyes and a cap of silver hair that frames her smooth Mediterranean skin. Her lips protrude slightly, suggesting that she is ready for a kiss. One could easily imagine her staring up at her husband with the silken gaze that elevates a man in his own eyes to the rank of world-class lover.

Except that Kalli did not have sex with her husband for the last fifteen of their forty years of marriage. When the fires ebbed—and they had never burned much beyond room temperature—she tried to reignite them. She has an indelible memory of the night she brought home a red lace nightgown. She dabbed on perfume and paraded past her husband, who was reading in bed. He looked up briefly and said, "That's the silliest thing I've ever seen."

I first interviewed Kalli over brunch. She is five feet two inches tall, very slender and shapely, with a tiny waist, which she accentuates by wearing torso-hugging silk shirts. She replayed a long-ago love affair that had begun on a drive from Chicago to the East Coast to start college. She, her brother, and Dylan, a handsome young Irishman who would become her brother's roommate at Yale, got a gig driving a hearse across the country. The three of them crowded together on the front bench seat, laughing and smoking Marlboros, rocking to the music of Chubby Checker, and swooning to Ray Charles's "I Can't Stop Loving You." Of course, Kalli and Dylan fell rapturously in love.

Kalli was confined in a women's junior college that felt to her like reform school, but she and Dylan kept up their romance by sheer ingenuity. Kalli drove down to Yale for weekends whenever she could, and they broke the rules to stay together in his room. "We did everything but intercourse, because of the fear of pregnancy," she recalls. "My Greek father would have killed me if I came home pregnant."

But Kalli's few joyful trespasses weren't enough to keep her from making the call that every college student makes at some point or other: "I can't stand it here anymore, I want to come home!" Her father welcomed the idea. Six months after Kalli went home to Chicago, where she floundered without a degree or a decent job prospect, she met a man ten years older who proposed to her.

"This will solve my life" was her only thought. Kalli's mother had been crushed by the lack of opportunities for traditional women, become an alcoholic, and died in her fifties from cirrhosis of the liver. Marriage offered Kalli the safety and permission to have sex. She threw herself into full-time homemaking, gardening, cooking, raising children—"and deferring," she added pointedly. "My inclination is to please people."

What was missing?

"I, uh, guess I created a story of what I wanted my life to be," she stammered. "We had a perfect family, wonderful children, we had a business together, a nice boat—and a very empty marriage. Our sex life probably ended in my thirties."

At 58, Kalli was seriously considering leaving her marriage. "I wouldn't want to be married again" was her definitive statement at this stage. "I've gotten used to living independently." She explained that she had become comfortable traveling alone, hiking and skiing alone, dining alone—and after all, she had always operated a small business on her own. "Because I was in an unhappy marriage, I had to learn to make my own happiness."

Kalli didn't expect that if and when she left that unhappy marriage, she would find a new lover. But just in case, she said, "I keep myself alive, sexually, with BOB."

Who's Bob? I asked.

"My battery-operated boyfriend."

After sharing a good laugh, I ask Kalli if she is comfortable having her intimate revelations in print. She says she is happy to tell her sexual story for the book, "because I know there are so many women out there who are suffering and who need to know it's okay to use a vibrator or erotica to keep yourself alive sexually if it's not happening with your partner."

Her friend Elizabeth was stunned when Kalli called her to confess that she was considering breaking out of her marriage. As a last resort, Kalli said, she and her husband had launched a massive renovation of their apartment. She went to great lengths to reassure her friend that she was not in pain. What she yearned for more than anything else was to live alone.

Taking a Leap into Lust

This attitude was foreign to Elizabeth. After divorcing and steeping herself in the study of Greek antiquities, she had made a deliriously happy second marriage with a sports buff. Her life had become very physical; they were always off skiing or sailing—until the day her husband died unexpectedly at the age of 57. For the two years after her husband's fatal heart attack, Elizabeth had been frozen in grief and fear. She was suddenly fully independent for the first time in her life, "but it was a *free-falling* independence." Elizabeth admitted to Kalli that she felt the cold tick-tock of the aging clock: "I really want to find a male partner before I dry up!"

Kalli had earlier come across a Yale alumni magazine at her brother's house. She was intrigued to read about her old boyfriend, Dylan, who was married and prospering in his own business in London. In a friendly gesture, she had e-mailed Dylan, and for the past several years they had kept up a casual correspondence. Then, the week before 9/11, Dylan let Kalli know that his marriage was over and he was moving to downtown New York. He was badly shaken by the breakup and the move. The shroud of smoke rising from Ground Zero only blocks from his new apartment made the window between retirement and death look to him as if it were closing fast.

Elizabeth had just decided that she was ready to venture into the uncertain waters of the over-60 dating pool when Kalli hit upon the idea of putting the two lonely hearts into e-mail contact. "I thought I was doing both of them a good deed," Kalli told me.

"But Dylan's your old boyfriend," Elizabeth protested. "I can't get involved with him."

"Elizabeth, please, I haven't seen him in almost forty years. But I've seen photos, so I know he still looks pretty good. Are you interested?"

"Absolutely."

After one ho-hum date, Elizabeth and Dylan went off traveling in different directions. But when they both ended up in New York again and he came to her hotel room, "It was just this instant take, bells and whistles went off, we could hardly make it from the sofa to the bedroom." That was how Elizabeth described to Kalli the idyllic weekend she and Dylan had spent together. The encounter was a jump start to a whole different concept of her future life. After two cold, celibate years, Elizabeth was astonished at how quickly the spark she felt with Dylan had inflamed her. Another few dates, and she invited him to spend a week with her in Chicago.

Kalli was surprised to receive an e-mail from Dylan: "Elizabeth wants to bring me to Chicago. She hopes we can meet you and your husband. Please say yes so we can all get together." Kalli invited the couple to stop by for a drink and see the apartment she and her husband had newly renovated.

That evening, after some initial awkwardness, Kalli's husband made a fire and they all sat in a cozy den and chatted about their various travels like polite strangers at a cocktail party. Dylan scarcely looked at Kalli, although he didn't seem terribly interested in Elizabeth either. Baffled by his impartiality, Kalli carried off her well-practiced charade of the perfectly ripened marriage.

Elizabeth's lusty affair with Dylan continued for the next couple of months, lifting her out of the misery of widowhood, but also reminding her of the adolescent highs and lows that a sexual relationship can bring—even to a postmenopausal woman. "I felt this teenage hormonal rush. It was like being thirteen again, that same level of anxiety. But my behavior was totally inappropriate for a sixty-year-old woman. I wrestled with questions like 'Is it worth it if I have to live with such a high anxiety level? And do I really want to accommodate to someone else's schedule?' "

While Elizabeth was dithering, she was caught short by receiving a "Dear John" letter from Dylan: "I find myself, miraculously, at my age, falling in love again," he wrote. "I would tell you the story, but it's too strange to be believed."

Just as she had anticipated, Elizabeth suffered the overwrought angst of a jilted adolescent. She phoned Kalli to complain, "I've lost Dylan to another woman—I think he's having a romance with a cocktail waitress in Big Sur."

Two months later, Kalli could not live with the guilt a minute longer. "Elizabeth," she confessed, "*I* am the other woman."

Rekindling the Old Flame

The magnetism between two people who were once in love, or even just young and infatuated, is so often able to hold its charge for decades—despite distance, marriages, births, divorces, and the dimming of more prosaic memories. That's why a woman will instinctively flinch when her husband's high school sweetheart just happens to call.

It was probably inevitable. That night in Chicago, in front of the fire Kalli's husband had lit, both she and Dylan had been reinfected by the sweet sickness of love, which had obviously lingered in both their systems for forty years. When Kalli listened to Elizabeth recount her amorous evenings with Dylan, it stirred envy and a long-suppressed desire. She had eventually summoned the nerve to send an e-mail to Dylan, telling him that she was getting a divorce. "I knew if I mentioned that, it would open up a door. But then I decided, 'What the hell! For forty years I've been such a good girl.' "

Dylan arranged to meet Kalli. They both knew the moment they hugged and said hello that Dylan would be spending the night with her.

"I was so anxious before you and Elizabeth came over for drinks that night," Kalli confessed. "I felt like I was sixteen and going out on my first date. But I tried as hard as I could not to look interested in you."

"You fooled me," he told her. "I couldn't look at you, either, or everybody would have known what I was thinking." He confessed that he still felt just like in the Ray Charles ballad "I Can't Stop Loving You."

Kalli began commuting to New York to spend every weekend she could with the long-lost love of her life. "The first thing it did for me, at the age of sixty, is to completely awaken my sexuality," she told me. "I knew I was multiorgasmic, but only with BOB. It's so much richer with a live man who you love! What I realized is that the sexual part of me is such an important part. I think about being with Dylan all the time, and look forward to it. I notice now that men are reacting differently to me. I'm not really coming on to them, so I don't know if it's the pheromones or what, but I have obviously become sexually attractive to other men as well."

This is so often the case. Women who are actively dating or in a romantic frame of mind, like Kalli—or Bebe the Oakland entertainer who, once she began dating after divorce, felt as if she had a neon sign on her forehead blinking "Available"—must send out some sort of signal. It serves as a reminder that any seasoned woman who is single should date as often as she can, even if it means enduring some dull evenings and disappointments.

For six months, Kalli kept telling herself that she was perfectly content to continue their relationship as a commuter romance. "I really didn't want to live with him," she told me, protesting a little too vigorously. "I wanted to hold on to my independence." But there was ultimately no denying that she and Dylan had found their soulmates. The more time they spent together, the more emotionally attached they were becoming. Kalli felt herself changing, softening. Since she and her husband had already agreed to an amicable divorce, she quickly arranged to sell her business and the big apartment on Lake Shore Drive with all its antiques. She invested her share of the proceeds and took an eight-hundred-square-foot one-bedroom rental apartment a few blocks from Dylan's Manhattan co-op.

"I couldn't be happier or more excited," she e-mailed me. "I love being with Dylan whenever we want, and I still have my independence."

In our last conversation, we marveled together at how far American women of our vintage have come in our evolution, as compared with women like Kalli's mother, who lived in a traditional, male-dominated marriage, never found herself, retreated into alcoholism, and died in her early fifties. Here was Kalli, now in her early sixties, fully alive and exhilarated about a whole new chapter in her life.

A Platonic Soulmate

Elizabeth's story was not finished, either. At a dinner party (after her husband's death but before Dylan) she had met a retired surgeon who traveled to many of the places she did in the quest for antiquities. Graham had invited her to dinner, but his approach had been rather abrupt; he asked, "How would you feel, if you found the right partner, about cohabitation?" Elizabeth was equally blunt: "I had an extraordinarily wonderful partnership and marriage, and I'm not expecting to find that again."

They didn't see each other again for a year.

In retrospect, Elizabeth realizes that she just wasn't ready. But months after she and Dylan split, she included Graham on an invitation list for a cocktail party she was throwing to help Kalli's lonely husband meet someone new. He was delighted to come. She and Graham began sneaking out to the movies in the afternoon, a delicious vagrancy available only to retired seniors with no pressing obligations to anyone else in the world. "It was clear to me that he was pursuing me as a friend," says Elizabeth, "but I didn't know if he was pursuing me as a sexual interest." He later told Elizabeth he had seen her as untouchable, and, frankly, intimidating. But once, at the movies, during a violent scene, Elizabeth reached over and grabbed Graham's upper arm. He grasped her hand, tightly, and didn't let go until the movie was over. Parting that evening, he told her, "When your hand touched my arm, an electric shock went right through me." He gave her a long, serious kiss.

They planned a weekend trip to New York for the opening of the renovated Museum of Modern Art. Graham had booked separate rooms at the Four Seasons. A few days before they left, Elizabeth called him and said, "I think it's silly for you to pay for two rooms."

They became lovers, and emerged as a couple within their social group in Chicago. They didn't live together, but he often slept over. He'd say, "I don't understand it. This is just not like me. I've not wanted to be around somebody the way I want to be with you for many, many years."

Later that year they took a cruise together. The sex was erratic. After spending a solid month in each other's company, they determined that 24/7 was too much time together. Their physical relationship ended, but another possibility opened up.

Once both Elizabeth and Graham let sexual expectations drop, they were able to form an intimate friendship as partners traveling through life, which seems to suit both of them at their age and stage. They have since traveled all over Europe and Asia together. And when they travel, they still sleep in the same room, in the same bed. They still cuddle. They just don't expect or ask for sex. Graham seems more relaxed, and Elizabeth surmises that he feels relief that he carries no romantic responsibilities.

"I'm happy with the relationship as it is now, because we can travel together or just go to movies together, we enjoy so many of the same things," says Elizabeth. "At a certain point I think it's okay to hang up the sex part. I find our relationship to be totally unique. But that is not to say I wouldn't welcome another sexual partner in the future."

Kalli and Elizabeth, by the way, continue to be fast friends. "We understand each other and what we most value at this stage in life," says Elizabeth. "I'm glad that Kalli has reconnected with the man she was probably meant for, and she knows what I've found out about myself. I'm hanging on to my independence for all it's worth."

❖   ❖   ❖

While it may be surprising for a woman to settle into a loving attachment with a soulmate—without sex—it is hardly unique. It's what the author-psychiatrist Dr. Ethel Person describes as "affectionate bonding." This is not infrequently what remains of a love affair after the passionate attraction fades. Or it can develop a life of its own in a friendship that never became sexual but always provided warmth, affection, tenderness, and nurturance. "When we compare love without sex to a more prevalent and commonly sanctioned alternative—the preservation of perfunctory sex within an emotionally depleted union—the former compromise may look very good indeed," writes Dr. Person. In marriages where the desire or capacity for sex most likely will not be revived, usually due to medication or the illness of one partner, affectionate bonding is often a satisfactory resolution.

As I stated much earlier, the most precious element of romantic love is making a real connection with a person who "gets you," and sees you in your best light. Both Kalli and Elizabeth have found soulmates with whom they share that connection. One includes a vivid sexual attraction. The other, by exempting sex, has allowed Elizabeth and Graham to forge for themselves an attachment rich with meaning, and a mutual commitment to remain soulmates for each other.

Chapter 23

Love Tested by Fire

"We have cancer."

"What kind of cancer?" the psychologist asked.

"Breast cancer," he said.

"Thank God I didn't ask him *who* had cancer, because that would have destroyed the beautiful shared identity he has developed with his wife," says Dr. Judith Wallerstein. The psychologist recognized this couple as being among those she identified in her research as having a good marriage in middle life, because when confronted by a major life crisis, they are handling it beautifully and it is bringing them closer together.

Seasoned women and men are all too likely at some point to be confronted by serious illness, or the loss of an identity-defining job. When such a dramatic setback intrudes on the life we take for granted, it affects the spouse as much as the wounded partner. On top of dealing with the uncertainties of survival—physically, financially, vocationally—there is an even more fearsome emotional doubt. We all hope and want our significant other to "love me for me." *But what if I'm down and out? What if I've lost my job—will I end up in a seedy furnished room, alone? What if I have breast cancer and the chemo makes me fat and bald? What if I don't feel like making love while I'm so weak—will you still love me?* How else to explain the broad popularity of the song recorded by the Beatles in 1967, "When I'm 64"? It was written by John Lennon and Paul McCartney when they were only in their mid-twenties, yet everybody could relate because everybody harbors those fears.

The possibilities for deepening the shared identity between you and your partner, however, are greatly heightened under duress—provided there was already a strong attachment. Those feelings may have been overshadowed by the petty vicissitudes of daily life, but when a crisis hits, if there is a wellspring that you can tap into, battling illness or unemployment together can produce moments of the deepest soul connection. A soulmate is uniquely suited to reading the emanations of his or her partner's soul and caring for them. This is the gift of a truly seasoned marriage or long-standing relationship.

A psychotherapist I interviewed was frank in saying that otherwise, caregiving can be a bitter pill. One patient revealed that when his wife was in great physical difficulty, he was having a very hard time being responsive to her. He was quite honest. "You know, the problem is, the bells never rang for us," he said. "When I go back over our courting and our early marriage, times the bells should have rung, it was never there. It was a marriage between two comrades and friends, but we never had a deeper connection." When his wife got better, he divorced her and found someone else.

When the Hammer Falls

It used to be the young and arrogant, on the lower rungs of the corporate ladder, who were first to be laid off during an economic downturn. Now it's the older, accomplished people, in their fifties and consigned to a seat at Starbucks with a laptop and cell phone, making cold calls. The men and women at greatest risk belong to the leading edge of the baby-boomer generation, who in 2006 are between the ages of 51 and 60, and are faced with the cruel prospect of being involuntary early retirees. Nipping at their heels are men and women of the "Me Generation," born from 1956 to 1965, who often have more advanced education and electronic savvy than their senior counterparts. Today, one fifth of the CEOs of the Standard & Poor's 500 companies are under the age of 50. At the same time, the percentage of CEOs who are 60 and older is decreasing.

James Atlas writes candidly in his book *My Life in the Middle Ages: A Survivor's Tale* about the dark night of the soul he entered when he was fired at 50. Suddenly dispatched from his lofty position as a senior editor at a Condé Nast publication, he describes the eerie silence in his boss's office and the panic clawing at his throat. He needed to get up and leave, but all he could think of was the tragic hero of Arthur Miller's *Death of a Salesman,* Willy Loman, on the day he was fired. Willy wouldn't leave the boss's office until the man finally excused himself and said, "Willy, I gotta see some people. Pull yourself together."

James admits that his heart had no longer been in the job he'd lost, and it had shown. This is common among men and women in their mid- to late fifties who grow weary of the competitive jockeying and incestuous politics of corporate life. But it's painful and financially frightening to be fired from a job where one thought one could coast. And many involuntary retirees in this age group won't be able to land a comparable position in their field, even though they have been successful. They are faced with having to live off their retirement savings ten to fifteen years before they expected to retire. Many men of James's age and generation are stunned at how early the ax is falling on them and their contemporaries—before they have even internalized that they are in middle life and need a new dream. I see a new law of natural selection operating among boomer men:

Men are living longer, but they're being replaced earlier.

Some men who are junked prematurely seem to wind down and die of a broken heart. This is particularly true of men I have observed who do not have a deep and loving partnership with a mate, but who have a utilitarian and emotionally distant relationship with a spouse and probably with their adult children. Every ounce of passion and ambition has been pumped into their careers. When that inflated ego is suddenly withdrawn from the constant power source of high position—deferential subordinates, expense account lunches, speedily returned phone calls, press clips, and perhaps most important, a place to go outside the home—there isn't much left for life support. Even if a wife has been sensitive and supportive, a man may not believe he is still worthy in her eyes. A wise senior psychologist in Berkeley, Dr. Hilda Kessler, has concluded from her work with many such men and their spouses that "men don't get the part in the marriage vows about 'the worse.' They get 'the better,' but not 'the worse,' until they're there. It's very common. They believe, 'You love me because I take care of you, because I bring home the bacon, because I do this or that, but if I'm unable to perform these tasks, I'm afraid you will no longer be attached to me, because I will no longer have a value to you.' It's only when a man is actually in a vulnerable situation and a spouse is supportive and nonjudgmental that it sinks in. There she is, being attentive, helpful, suggesting new ways of thinking about his future, and he may come to realize it couldn't be because of his instrumental value, because his instrumental value is on hold at this time. Hopefully, it will eventually dawn on the man, 'It must be me.' "

Forced early retirees who have talent and drive, a supportive working spouse, and some cash—if they can let go of the need to be defined by a corporate identity—may find that being shot out of a cannon lights their fire again. It's a chance to become more entrepreneurial, to buy or start their own business. James Atlas not only landed on his feet, he found multiple avenues for his talents as a magazine writer and author. He also began to commission and publish his own extensive collection of short biographies of famous figures.

For Better or Worse

I learned about the kind of bond a life crisis can forge more than ten years ago, when a growth previously dismissed as benign was found to be cancerous. My husband's first words to me when we learned his diagnosis set the tone for all that was to come: "Don't worry. We'll get through this together." At his insistence, we continued with our plans for the evening and enjoyed a gala concert at the New York Philharmonic. But the next morning, it was still true. We had cancer. It had lodged in my husband's body, but it threatened the very fabric of both of our lives. Armored by our long and loving partnership in life, we got down in the trenches side by side, mere grunts facing a stealthy foe that never shows its face. Our weapons were faith, hope, and love. The greatest of these is love.

Our faith we put in God and in the medical professionals, whom we chose with great care, not only for their known expertise but for the "click" of intuitive recognition we felt with doctors who connected with us personally and had a human touch. One such man was Dr. John Connolly, a renowned New York surgeon who had pioneered a procedure that minimized disfigurement. He taught and practiced at both St. Vincent's and Columbia-Presbyterian Hospitals, and had an array of young disciples, but the word was that nobody had the hands of the artist like the artist himself. We asked to see Dr. Connolly.

A tall, white-haired man with a gentle face and discerning eyes greeted us like old friends. After he had done a thorough examination and expressed a jaunty confidence in the outcome of treatment, he could see that we were still hesitating to leave. We didn't have to ask about his age—he volunteered.

Sitting knee to knee with us in his consulting room, his old-school golfing knickers peeking from beneath his lab coat, Dr. Connolly extended his long, sensitive fingers. "I'm eighty-one years old, but I still do three of these surgeries a week, and they last from four to five hours." He held his hands stock still for probably a full minute. In that minute, we all felt a silent affirmation that beneath the superficial vulnerabilities of age or infirmity, people may have strengths beyond measure.

"But if you're still worried, let me know," said the surgeon with sincere humility.

We responded, almost in unison, "We have great confidence in you, Doctor."

He then invited us to seal the bond of mutual need for reassurance: "I will ask of you only one thing. On the morning of the surgery, I want you to tell me, 'You're going to do a splendid operation.' "

We had gone to Dr. Connolly's office to take the measure of his competence, but what we came away with was a measure of his soul. On the way out, we learned that not only was he an artist with the scalpel, he was an artist at heart. He gave us one of the eight books of poetry he'd written on weekends.

Soaring with hope based on this confident second opinion, we emerged into the splurge of April sunshine and the boldness of leaves unfolding in the pear trees above us. The world was new again. My husband suddenly grabbed me and right on the street swept me into a full-frontal kiss. He was flooded with the juices of life and elixir of hope. The years fell away.

The surgery went splendidly, but the first look at the love of your life after a major operation is a shattering moment. Coming into my husband's hospital room and seeing him hooked up to a dizzying array of tubes and lines, his face slackened by drugs, his throat sprouting an apparatus that would temporarily breathe for him, it was hard to find a piece of him that still looked human and alive. I found his hand. Squeezed it. And from somewhere in the recesses of consciousness, he registered my touch. His hand squeezed mine back. It was the most exquisite moment. Beyond words. Just the touching of two souls. A fusion of love and shared hope. I knew the rest was going to be fine.

It's at the end of treatment that the fears rush in. This is very often when a cancer patient slides into depression. It may seem paradoxical and baffle the patient's family, but it is entirely understandable. While the patient is fully engaged in the daily struggle of treatment, with his medical team cheering him on, his family being aggressively supportive, and friends shoring him up, there is a great sense of momentum. But once his medical warriors have done all they can, he is left hanging. There is no clear outcome; nothing more to do but wait and see. Marking time until the six-month visit, the year-end test, and the subsequent visits and tests, which continue more or less indefinitely.

If the central motivator of all human activity is passion, its opposite is depression. This is the absence of vitality, when all the emotional color in life drains and one is left in darkness, or, worse, the void. Soul is absent. Faith is absent. God is absent. Depression can be contagious. It can infect the constant caregiver like a flu of the personality. One feels helpless to pull the sufferer back from the dark. The natural instinct is to cheerlead: "Hey, it's a beautiful day out there, why don't you take a walk and enjoy the sunshine!" That only plunges the depressed person more deeply into despair. Even if he did take that walk, he wouldn't feel the sun or smell the flowers, and that would intensify his sense of the void.

What I found was most appreciated was the simple act of massaging my husband's feet. Slowly. Toe by toe. I learned reflexology so I could pretend to myself I was doing something physically beneficial—and maybe I was—but the real benefit was to be present with him through his suffering. Silently, for the most part. Being present and in touch, to keep him connected to the world of the living by this simple, tactile act. He would eventually fall asleep, looking blissful.

When a person comes out of depression, falls back into his soul, and reclaims his life, he may find a new core of spiritual understanding. He may at last be able to feel worthy of God's love, and that of others.

Strangers appeared in our path at the darkest moments to shine light in new directions; I thought of them as angels. Sharing faith in these divine interventions and sustaining hope with the help of our medical partners were both essential to recovery. But it was the third weapon in our arsenal that turned out to be the most vital of all. Being loved—and being able to accept love—is the best mode of healing. To my amazement, once we began the battle with cancer, I discovered that my husband didn't know this weapon was available, or even how to use it.

During a hiatus in his treatment, my husband and I went to see Dr. Lawrence LeShan, a research and clinical psychologist, considered one of the fathers of mind-body therapy and author of the landmark book *Cancer as a Turning Point.* He has studied and demonstrated how the immune system—the cancer-fighting defense—can often be rebuilt by regenerating a person's enthusiasm for life. He encouraged my husband "to focus not on what's wrong with you, but on what's right with you."

The most poignant revelation came when Dr. Ruth Bolletino, a psychotherapist who has trained and worked with Dr. LeShan, uncovered the fact that, despite the love that was pouring in from all sides, my husband wasn't receiving it. He believed the only reason people cared about him was for his instrumental value as an editor—what he could do for others in their careers. Although hundreds of people had sent him affectionate notes and commiserated with him, he had received them not as expressions of their regard for him as a person, but as their regret in being deprived of his role in potentiating them. What came out of the session was that he'd also felt that way about me. He'd never fully believed that I loved him *for him* and would be devoted to him no matter what. It came as a rude shock. We had been married by then for about ten years, and together off and on for many years before that.

◆   ◆   ◆

Once the battle against the beast picked back up again, we worked side by side to find the right doctors, choose the best postsurgical protocol, and assemble a solid support network. It was during this battle that my husband came to realize I *was* with him, sometimes so close it was as if we existed under the same skin—and it was because I loved him for him.

The role of the spouse in a situation such as this is one of caretaker of the soul. The medical team takes care of the body, and while the spouse must act as the patient's advocate and medical monitor, the even more important role of the caregiver is to keep the soul nourished—by just being there, offering good and healthy food, music, laughter, massage, foot rubs, and guided meditations, reading aloud, or listening to a book on CD together. And long and longer walks and talks.

If you ask most men when they're sick or scared, "How are you feeling?" you'll get the stock stoic monosyllable "Fine" or "Okay." You seldom get much information. When you are able to connect at the soul level, you become hyperaware of the signals the wounded partner sends. It's like someone who is very musical and able to hear notes that others might not pick up. Because you are so tuned in to each other, you pick up nonverbal signals. The verbal level is a secondary system—it's a telling about what is. But when two people connect on the "is" level, you're on the primary level. You don't need words. When you feel that soul connection with another person, that person feels it, too. I think that's what everybody is looking for in a committed relationship. It's not just love, it's love plus—a love that has been subdued by circumstance, tested and strained, but that keeps roaring back, stronger than ever.

When there was some doubt about whether to begin another regimen of debilitating treatment, "to be on the safe side," we were able to have a friendly consultation with another senior physician known worldwide for his contributions to cancer treatment, Dr. Morton Coleman. Dr. Coleman questioned my husband, not about his body but about what enlivened his mind. He then dispensed a booster of the best medicine of all, and it wasn't medical. It was the elixir of wisdom refined over thirty-five years of following his patients, pushing the envelope of research, and acting as clinical professor of medicine at New York Weill Cornell Medical Center and director of its Center for Lymphoma and Myeloma.

"Go out and live your life as fully as you know how!" commanded this expansive man in his boldly confident voice. "Change it, make it great, the two of you, together. That will do more for recovery than any further treatment." We did, and he was right.

My husband was gradually able to accept the fact that he can be loved even in a vulnerable state. It has been a realization not only of what he can receive, but also of what he can give to others. If a man wounded by life is able to express love to friends when they are down, when they have fallen through the career cracks or been laid low by a devastating diagnosis, he will find it easier to accept that others can feel love and compassion for him—in his rawness, in his originality, in the naked essence of himself.

Once found, this force of love that is discovered under extreme circumstances can grow and grow. It fortifies both partners against future crises. If you've been there together before, you both know you can return to that depth of attachment and that when you get there—even in the face of fear and illness—it can be blissful. My husband said to me during one such period, "Sometimes we're remarkably close in a way that is not everyday common. And those moments are not necessarily sexual—they're about things we did together, things we said, things we explored together. The times when you've saved my life, a whole physical flood of love immerses me."

Sustaining the Soul Connection Through Unspeakable Tragedy

I was particularly moved by the accommodation to tragedy devised by a midwestern woman who joined our group interview at the University of Minnesota. This was a group of seasoned women who had been married and divorced and, in their forties or fifties, had found their greatest love with older men to whom they were very much attached. When the conversation turned to the fickleness of sexual desire and the changing functional capacities of men after 60, a woman with a lilting Irish accent chimed in: "Don't I wish I were enjoying passionate sex with a lover, but there are many ways to have relationships that are intensely intimate, but not sexual."

Everyone turns to listen to Carol Connolly, a poet and local columnist who is well known and liked in her community. With her strawberry blond hair and ebullient personality, one would not guess she is just past 70. She is noticeably at ease in her own skin, which was evident when, despite a slight osteoporotic bend to her upper back, she glided into the room with a long cardigan sweater over Hepburn-style trousers and a black turtleneck.

This is a woman with eight children who dispatched her first husband several times before they found the courage to make their divorce stick; that's how bad the situation was. Her defense against despair was to begin writing wickedly funny free verse. She is a lusty woman, and cerebral pleasures went only so far in counteracting the chaos of playing Mother Goose to a houseful of fatherless kids. While divorcing, she met a composer and musician who had just the sort of quirky, creative personality that meshed with hers.

"I call him Boyfriend Bill," she says with a girlish smirk. "I swear that God sent him to me. He was a great friend to my children. And he absolutely fired me up sexually, not that those fires had died down."

Carol lived with Boyfriend Bill at a time when she still had a couple of kids at home. Both carried too many wounds from their divorces to want to risk legally formalizing their relationship. "But we were more 'married' than I was to my actual former husband," she says. "We shared everything. Bill was a brilliant, creative, absolutely charming man, bighearted and just plain big—six feet, five inches and three hundred pounds—and he looked invulnerable." One day he finished a script for a play and went off to New York to meet potential backers. On the corner of Ninety-fifth Street, a car plowed into him. His head exploded through the driver's windshield. The driver punched the bloody head right back out so he could speed off.

The rest of the story Carol relates with toneless restraint: "He was in a coma for a month. We flew him home by air ambulance, and he was in a variety of hospitals for a year before I brought him home. But he has a severe brain injury, and I couldn't care for him."

That awful tragedy was ten years ago. She was 61. "It took me a long time to realize, to accept, that he's really damaged," she admits. It was several years before she could acknowledge that "this is not the same person. I mean, his core is the same, but the man I knew is never coming back."

Girding herself with her antic sense of humor, she began referring to him as "my brain-injured Boyfriend Bill." She had herself named his court-appointed guardian and tried out a variety of living situations for him, finally settling on an adult foster care home. Despite Bill's loss of short-term memory, and the erasure of any boundaries between his waking and dream life, they can still talk and laugh and cherish their shared history.

"Writing is what has helped me keep my sanity," she tells us. Carol has had two books of humorous verse published and has nearly finished a third. But she isn't ready, at 71, to be sentenced to emotional and sexual death for life. Her younger friends keep fixing her up with their fathers, who are her age and usually widowed. "I've had a few hilarious dates," she says, launching into the story about the appellate judge who was great fun on their first dinner date but not exactly a long-term prospect. "He got home and went immediately into a nursing home—he's still there!" Another blind date brought her together with a beefy Irishman. He had one topic of conversation, his dead wife—who had already been in the grave for five years. Carol finally said, "You know, I've had a little tragedy in my life, too." She never heard from him again.

"But I have to say, my brain-injured Boyfriend Bill is more interesting than most men in my age group. He hasn't lost his basic brilliance, his way of dissecting a problem, and the positive philosophy he brings to it. He can still help me sort out little problems. I might say, 'Oh, I did a reading of my poems today, and in the Q&A afterwards I gave the dopiest answer.' He'll say, 'You're always entertaining, I'm sure people liked it.' "

Carol had recently spent two weeks in Palm Desert, California, in a time-share condo where she was invited to a cocktail hour that turned out to be a singles over-50 event. Finding it both hilarious and disheartening, she made careful mental notes so she could later phone Bill and regale him with her descriptions. "There was enough silicone in the room to launch a space capsule," she told him. "I met a surgically improved woman who was looking for a sixth husband and a new mortgage at a lower rate, whichever came first." Boyfriend Bill hooted with delight.

"I guess this means I may be lost to new romance, at least for now," Carol tells us. "But my Bill is the best friend I've ever had. I love being with him, and then I'm very happy to take him to his home at the end of the night."

The poet's love life is far from complete, but she does have the sustaining base of a soulmate—a depth of connection that could hardly be reproduced with anyone else at this stage—and by dating occasionally, she diversifies her male company. More important, her family and her work give her a structure and a lively built-in social life. "I have eleven grandchildren, and because I write a gossip column for a Minnesota magazine, I get invited everywhere," Carol continues. "And I have my poetry. I personally think for women like me, or most of you, our lives are very full." The other women murmur their assent. "But if someone came along, I'd be open to it."

What would she be looking for in a man at this stage?

She muses, "It might be nice to have a driver." Suddenly the mischievous gleam reappears in her eyes; she has another story. "I ran into an old friend of my mother's who is now about eighty-five. I said, 'How are you, Mrs. Bliss?' She said, 'Oh, I'm not Mrs. Bliss any longer, dear. I'm remarried.' She leaned in and deadpanned, 'I had to. You know, dear, I don't drive.' "

Part VI

Graduating to Grandlove

*G*randlove is the payoff phase in the arc of pursuing the passionate life. I asked couples to compare the marriages or love relationships they have developed in their Second Adulthood to those in their earlier life. Their responses revealed a softening of the sharper edges of anger, conflict, blaming, bullheadedness, and self-absorption, and a rise in self-confidence and self-control. With a greater acceptance of their differences, they enjoy the bonus of greater spontaneity. Here are some typical descriptions of grandlove from my respondents in their sixties and seventies.

"I feel more calm, less stressed and distracted than when I was younger, so I have time to think things through and work them out without a fight."

"I don't feel the same need to get even as when I was young."

"I stand up for myself more now, and that applies to many older women I know."

"I'm more tolerant now, less the demanding, know-it-all guy I was in my earlier years."

"Marriage gets easier, my husband and I have more time to clear up a misunderstanding before it turns into a fight."

"My wife has become more spontaneous in the things we do together."

"My husband is more willing to join me in group activities I've always enjoyed."

A New York woman describes herself as a former adrenaline junkie who worked in the advertising business and went through a period of rabid feminism and two marriages before she hit her fifties. "I'm now fifty-eight and more tolerant," she says. "I'm more willing to let things go. It's such a relief. I don't have to solve that problem today."

These are not just random personality changes. Aging experts now appreciate that psychological growth and development continue throughout the life cycle. As we are tested by the vicissitudes of life, we have abundant opportunities to make midcourse and late-course adjustments.

Our neurochemistry also changes as we get older. There is a shift in the proportions of male and female sex hormones. The ratio of the "male" sex hormone, testosterone, to estrogen in a postmenopausal woman may be up to twenty times higher than in a woman who is still ovulating and making estrogen in her ovaries. The fact that a woman's Second Adulthood is fueled by a dominance of testosterone coincides with the resurgence in women of adventurousness, independence, and assertiveness.

In a man, as his testosterone levels lower with age, the ratio shifts in the opposite direction. In addition, more of his "male" sex hormone is converted into estrogen. It is not an abrupt change, and males will always have at least ten times as much testosterone as females. Some neurobiologists now speculate that our brains, bathed as they are in our hormones, actually change *structurally* in later life. This could be part of the reason men uncover more of their "feminine" side, and women their "masculine" side, in Second Adulthood.

You may have a cherished mate, an intimate friend, or a platonic partner, but at this stage in the arc of passionate living, that person does not have to be ever present in your life. The love may be just as deep and even more nurturing, but your relationship has probably matured. One or both of you may be restricted by health limitations. Or one of you may be much freer because of retirement from your job, while the other is still actively engaged in work or building a business. Grandlove means still maintaining a loving relationship, which may transcend the need to live or travel together all the time.

The Playful Side of Grandlove

Another kind of rebirth also happens for many women in the postmenopausal years. When we get the call from a daughter or daughter-in-law announcing that the first grandchild has begun to push into the world, the primal throb of fertility revs up again. (In my case, during my daughter's first pregnancy, I became "pregnant" with the writing of my first full-length play.) Vicariously, we women enjoy a second chance at mothering. And this time we're not on night duty, not juggling the pressures of young marriage together with career conflicts. We're the funsters; when the squalling starts at the end of the day, we can walk away.

The love that women and men feel for their grandchildren adds another whole dimension to middle and later life. Grandchildren are a carousel; riding a day with them is a return to total spontaneity and innocence, living in the moment, drinking it in with all the senses wide open and primed for surprises. We have full permission to bring back a playful side and indulge in the delights of each age. The floor-crawling, "I'm gonna getchoo" stage evolves into the sharing of a private language, as together you shape baby talk into words. There's the 2-year-old who lives so much in the present that every time you leave the room and return, he squeals "Hi!" as if it were a brand-new day. Then comes the first sleepover, where you and your little accomplice abandon table discipline and play spoons on glasses and dishes to accompany a CD with your own rhythm section. How great is it to be taught to drop-kick by a 3-year-old? To help him break in his first baseball mitt? To make whipped cream with a 4-year-old and let the beaters spatter it all over you and the kitchen while you revel in the child's ecstatic squeals?

Grandparenting is a rebirth that eases the pinch of boundaries closing in on our own brief existence. It offers us another chance to leave an imprint of love on the time after our time. Even Norman Thayer, the bitter "old poop" of the classic play and movie *On Golden Pond,* who on the eve of his eightieth birthday is obsessed with death and not quite fully present in life, is revived when a 13-year-old boy busts into his entropy and calls his bluff: "Are you bullshitting me?" Once Norman begins taking the kid fishing, the special bond that skips a generation begins forming between them. By the end of the play, Norman has a new reason to live—to visit the boy, now his new stepgrandchild, in California.

In the absence of a significant other, the love aspect may be sustained by drawing closer to other family members; and certainly by strengthening friendship networks with other women. People without their own grandchildren can find surrogates in grandnieces and -nephews, students or younger colleagues, in community "grandparenting," sports coaching, or literacy programs. But it is essential, in my view, that we connect with the future through relationships with the young people who will follow us.

The Transition to Wise Woman

Women who pursue a more passionate life, and continue to find sources of companionship and intimacy, accumulate the charms and powers of fully seasoned women. They learn acceptance of what they cannot change. They become more tolerant of others' differences and idiosyncrasies and more aware and confident of their own uniqueness.

If women take full advantage of their potential to develop greater strength in their fifties and sixties, they graduate into wise women. If they don't do it right, they can turn into foolish women. Those are the women we see running to get face-lifts that turn their countenance into marble, women who cling to their adult children because they have no other real life, or who keep telling you what they accomplished at 35 because there has been nothing much new since then.

Finding a partner, sexual or platonic, with whom to share the third age can happen anytime. True friendship may be the most lasting form of love, especially when the partners are committed to working together toward the same goal or cause, or thrive on pride in each other's contributions to family and society.

When we reach the mature years, most of us are looking for depth, for meaning, for value. We want it within our sexual lives, within our companionable lives, and with any person or any place where we might leave a mark. That way, when we reach Erikson's last stage of adulthood— Integrity or Despair—we can look back and say, yes, this life had worth, it was not an empty bag of wind "that passeth away as the remembrance of a guest that tarrieth but a day."

Transcendence

The Grandlove stage is also marked by the development of a "communal heart," when we are better able to leave our self-interest at the door and turn our love outward to envelop the surrounding community. Once our children are grown and gone, there is a renewed need for connection with others. This urge to reach out and give back is well illustrated by the ways in which women form networks to nurture and take care of one another in middle and later life.

Sooner or later, we all must face the reality that there will be an end. We are only too mortal, as the friends who pass on before us make painfully plain. The Grandlove phase coincides with the Passage to the Age of Unity on the ladder of adult development. It is essential that each of us come to a passion or a cause or a meaning or a dream that we hope might transcend our own passage out of this life. A realignment of our goals with a view toward what we will leave behind may lead us to transcendence in one of several ways:

We may create a sense of continuity through honest, inspirational relationships with our children and grandchildren. This is the love path.

We may create, or foster, some work that achieves symbolic immortality. This is the dream path, developed into a purpose and put into practice in the world.

We may act to promote good or eradicate bad in the world, which serves to ratify our own worth. This is the spiritual path in action.

Chapter 24

Later–Life Romances and Remarriage

*D*eep bonds of affection and respect grow like mature vines between couples who find each other in their Selective Sixties, Spontaneous Seventies, and later. Nursing homes are reporting that the fires of romance still burn between their elderly charges, who sometimes act more as though they were in junior high, with hot and heavy romances and breakups.

Enlightened American facilities are now training their staffs to stay cool if they catch two residents in the same bed, and not to be judgmental. Just because people are in a nursing home doesn't mean they can't have romantic or sexual feelings for someone else.

In the recent past, women rarely entered into marriage after the age of 50. Remarriages among women aged 50 to 75 made up only .5 percent of all marriages over the half century between 1925 and 1975, according to data from the U.S. Census Bureau. But by 1996, the census report reflected the boom in midlife romance and the rise of seasoned love, with women aged 45 to 64 accounting for almost 10 percent of all marriages. After women reach 65, however, the rush to remarry drops off: only 1 percent of marriages in 1996 involved women 65 years or older.

So how does it happen that two proud and proper widowed people, with a first lifetime already behind them, find each other in their midsixties and almost seamlessly craft a soul connection? Emily Anne's story illustrates that it's not too late to start the pursuit of yet another passionate life.

Pursuing Mr. Wonderful

"I'm so happy that you and Gedney found each other," a friend gushed. Word had gotten around that the widow Emily Anne Staples was about to be remarried to one of the most hotly pursued widowers in Minneapolis.

"We didn't," said Emily Anne. "I went after him."

When I asked Gedney how old he had been when he proposed to Emily Anne, he gave a self-deprecating groan. "Oh, my God, sixty-something."

"He was sixty-seven," Emily Anne offers proudly. "I was sixty-five."

"Had either of you ever thought, in your earlier life, that you would have a passionate love and marriage at that age?"

"Of course not!" Gedney retorted.

"It never occurred to me!" Emily Anne chimed in.

In her forties, the mother of four children, she had tossed her hat into the ring of state electoral politics. She went through most of the phases of pursuing a passionate life with her first husband. She followed her new career dream, learned how to live alone when she went to graduate school in another city, and learned the skills and adaptations that carry one through the aging process. Those rich experiences gave her the appetite and confidence not to retreat into widowhood in her mid-sixties and hang up her passions. On the contrary, when the opportunity presented itself to enter into a late Romantic Renaissance, she was ready to pounce.

Emily Anne never pictured herself without a good man at her side. All through her first marriage of more than thirty years—and a contented marriage it was—Emily Anne admits, "I'd kept my eye on Gedney." Embarrassed into honesty, Gedney says, "I think we both did." Through his two previous marriages, Gedney had held Emily Anne in his peripheral vision. She has never been shy, and even after being widowed in her late fifties, she continued to feel confident about herself as a sexual being; he noticed that. One can't miss her as she makes her way through a crowded restaurant; her broad smile and the slightly devilish lilt in her speech spell fun, and, indeed, she is invariably stopped by members of the political establishment to jawbone about city or state issues. She had approached Gedney now and then on fund-raising drives, and he had always been happy to make a modest contribution.

Somewhat facetiously, Emily Anne describes him as "a pickle packer." True enough, but Gedney Tuttle ranks among the pantheon of pickle packers; Gedney Pickles has been a manufacturing mainstay in the upper Midwest since 1880 and privately held by his family for six generations. What's more, Gedney still cuts a dashing figure in his sixties with his classic features and winter ski tan, set off by a nimbus of silver hair.

Emily Anne is a star in her own pantheon of Minnesota state politics. She has held political office at several levels. Her natural Irish political genes were honed by working with her father, a pioneer in the public relations field and a deputy mayor of Minneapolis. Had she graduated from the University of Minnesota with a later generation of women, Emily Anne probably would have resisted the family and social pressure to enter into marriage at 25; she was having much too good a time working in New York and gadding about Europe, pursued by a string of boyfriends. But that was the Fifties, and her parents maneuvered a good match for her with the scion of a fine old Minneapolis family. As a woman, and Catholic Democrat, marrying a man who was a Protestant Republican, Emily Anne subsumed her early political identity and worked tirelessly for the Republican Party, even as she produced four children.

In 1974, then in her forties, she bolted from the party. Her heart was in campaigning for the Equal Rights Amendment. When the state Republican leaders repudiated the ERA and a woman's right to choose, and with the party in disarray after the resignation of President Nixon, Emily Anne returned to her political roots. The Democrats immediately recognized her talents and approached her to run for public office. She lost her first contest as a Democrat, but in 1976 she swept into the state government as the first woman Democrat elected a Minnesota state senator.

"I celebrated my fiftieth birthday in the Senate cloakroom," she recalls. "It was fabulous!"

Not one to brood on her losses in life, when Emily Anne was defeated for reelection, she set out to become a student again. With her last child finishing high school, she moved to Cambridge, Massachusetts, for her fifty-second year to study at the John F. Kennedy School of Government. Learning to live alone would stand her in good stead.

The shock of losing her husband to a sudden heart attack when she was 59 was muted by the immediate demands of a campaign. At the time she was chairing a division of the United Way. She was able to alleviate some of her grief by focusing on public policy. "I was busy and feeling fulfilled. I didn't have to worry about getting home to make dinner. The children were, of course, on their own, so life was not bad." When she was elected to the county board, she started traveling all the time. "So I was definitely not at home pining."

❖   ❖   ❖

It's Valentine's Day eve, and I have the honor of being invited as a third wheel to the anniversary dinner marking the night, eleven years ago, when Gedney proposed to Emily Anne. What I want to know is, how did these two highly independent seniors find love, and how has it colored their passage into the Spontaneous Seventies?

The setting Gedney chose is winter romantic. They have a private room in a fashionable café, with a view of Loring Park misted in a light snowfall, tinged gold by turn-of-the-century streetlamps. Gedney orders a martini for himself and consults Emily Anne on the wine list. She demurs to his choice; this is a woman who knows instinctively how to let a man have his way when it doesn't really matter. Gedney decides we will share a bottle of Pinot Noir and indulge in a foie gras starter. Emily Anne's first words about her partner come in quick response to my question "Are you still a county commissioner?"

"Oh no, I retired when Mr. Wonderful came into my life."

Right there is clue number one. Apart from celebrity workaholics who prize fame, money, and power over personal relationships, many women who have advanced to prestigious positions in corporate life, law, medicine, or politics step back on the brink of going for the top leadership spot. They see the sacrifice it takes to be a CEO or managing partner or chief of service or, as in Emily Anne's case, a county supervisor who is traveling all the time. They know they will be largely isolated. As the boss, one can't be real friends with subordinates, or with competitors, and there isn't much time left over to revitalize a midlife marriage, expand a network of friends, or cultivate a soulmate if one should be fortunate enough to have the chance.

Intuitively, I believe, women are less obsessed with holding on to external power as they get older. They know that one day, in the cold light of dawn, they'll be replaced. This is the point when many women decide to start a business of their own, building on their know-how and contacts and enjoying discretionary power over how much time they devote to work, and when. What would they have left if an obsession with power and position undermined their marriage, or estranged them from their adult children, and prevented them from bonding with their grandchildren? Would they later regret being left out of the string of women friends who were becoming tighter, all the while the female CEO was running numbers on a company that will scarcely notice her absence?

Once Emily Anne made up her mind that she and Gedney had the potential to become soulmates, she surprised her political cronies. They were urging her to run for reelection to the county board and promising that she would be named chairman. Gedney was fully supportive.

"I told you I could handle that, didn't I?" He looks at Emily Anne.

"You told me that, but I realized there are limits to tolerance," she says. "It was far more important to me to start our life together, and not to be running off for early-morning meetings and late-evening meetings. It would have divided me."

In our sixties, we have to be selective. The dividedness that is unavoidable in earlier stages, when career building and family raising are constantly in competition, is no longer an imperative. Emily Anne was clear about her choice. I ask if she worried about letting go of that important part of her life.

"No, I didn't," she says with a serene smile. "I made a terrific trade." She has continued to be very active in health care policy as a volunteer in state and local organizations.

Gedney stops the dialogue to ask Emily Anne, "Are you enjoying the foie gras?" She murmurs and puckers up as he spoons another morsel between her lips.

I ask Gedney if he knew Emily Anne when they were younger. "I was one of her many dates in college." He turns to her for verification. "Did we actually meet on the Psi U front lawn?" She nods. Gedney adds, "Nothing ever serious."

Emily Anne interjects, "I was dating Hank."

"I thought she was very attractive," Gedney says. When I ask him to describe what she looked like, the shades of seminal memory pull down and shut out the intervening fifty years: "She looked about what she looks like now. A devastating smile that would knock your socks off."

Emily Anne strokes in the detail: "I had flowers in my hair. I'd been dating somebody who sent me flowers every Monday."

Gedney's rivalrous spirit immediately surfaces: "He was a real jerk."

"But his taste in flowers was splendid," says Emily Anne coyly.

"As was his taste in women."

The flirtatious banter between these two septuagenarians is testimony to the fact that it's never too late to enjoy romantic love. Another clue to their success at last-chance love is chemistry. It flared first more than fifty years ago, simmered through their respective marriages, and reignited at a much higher boil once they were both widowed. As stated earlier, if there is chemistry at the start of a relationship, it offers a built-in insulation against the assaults of aging, boredom, and unpredictable life crises. This pair also has a common history of time and place. And since they are age-appropriate for each other, they share a common vision of what they want for the future.

As the crown roast of lamb is served with a flourish, oozing juices, I ask the couple to describe how they reconnected. Emily Anne has no reservations about admitting "I had three men that I thought, 'If anything ever happens to their wives, I'll make a move.' "

Gedney leans forward. "I don't want to know who the other two are."

"You'll never know."

When Emily Anne read his wife's obituary in the newspaper, she lost no time in writing a condolence note to Gedney. He says, "I decided that part of the recovery process in grieving is to keep busy, so I responded with notes to every one of the condolences, one of which was Emily Anne's."

That gave her the opening to write a follow-up note, expressing her understanding of how he felt, having gone through the same thing, and tossing out a casual invitation to go to the movies sometime. I ask him if he received many such notes. He says he doesn't remember any but Emily Anne's.

Six weeks after her second note, Gedney called her up on a Sunday afternoon to see a movie. Again, he explains his move as part of a pre-scriptive program for getting through grieving: "I was told it's good health not to be alone." Emily Anne followed up with an invitation to go bicycling, and then to a football game with seats on the fifty-yard line and a pregame luncheon. Gedney flushes with pleasure at the memory of being courted. "She was pretty aggressive."

"I was a brazen hussy!" Emily Anne blurts out. But she reminds him that he was cooperating. After a couple of months of seeing each other, Emily Anne invited Gedney to be her escort at the inauguration of the new mayor of Minneapolis. Saying good night, Gedney ventured into her front hall and gave her a passionate kiss. A few days later, Gedney came by to pick her up for dinner but suggested instead that they buy some fresh fish and eat at home.

Emily Anne laughs. "The fish turned out to be old and terrible." But Gedney got a cozy fire going in the library, and Emily Anne brought a quilt down from the bedroom to cover the floor.

"And we snuggled."

"That was when sunshine came into my life," says Gedney.

A few weeks later they were having lunch at a department store and discussing the possibility of putting their lives together. To seal their intentions, they bought a quilt. "It was a terrible quilt." This time Gedney laughs. "But I did want us to spend the rest of our lives together, and I suppose buying that quilt was a gesture of commitment."

What was his inner image of himself at that time, in his late sixties? I ask Gedney.

"About thirty-five. I've never had a problem with whatever age I am."

"I think he's very sexy," offers Emily Anne.

"Oh, God, you don't have to go into *that.*"

"I just want to say that you made me feel very much like a woman again."

A month later, on Valentine's Day, Gedney formally proposed. He continued as CEO of the family company, but four years later he reconsidered the priorities in his life. "I figured that seventy-two might be a good time to retire. There were changes that needed to be made in the company, and I didn't have much interest in making them. I had two sons who were interested in taking over. I'm just as busy now as I was then, only I'm not getting paid."

Only in retrospect did I do the math and realize that they are in their late seventies now, yet neither one wore glasses or had trouble hearing or walking. They have remodeled a house to enclose their new life together. It sits on Lake Minnetonka, and they often take their little boat for a spin before sunset and enjoy a cocktail on the water. They make it a point to have dinner together every night. The most cherished time is cuddling in the morning before they have breakfast together, looking out and waiting for the sun to spill over the edge of the lake. But theirs is no sedentary existence. The day after our dinner they were flying to New York to walk Christo's gates in Central Park, take in a couple of plays, and then fly to Montana to go skiing at Big Sky.

Never Too Late

Even the hardest cases among divorcées who fill their middle years with high-profile careers may be startled by a sudden change of heart in their sixties. Rollene Saal is a prime example. Well known and respected in the New York publishing world as a smart, assertive, senior editor at one major publishing house after another, for many years she held the influential position of editor in chief of a major book club. At the time of her divorce, she had three small children, plus her influential job. She became consumed with her career and remained single for most of her adult life. Always turned out in a stylish business suit and spiky heels, Rollene did everything in a New York minute. She was friendly but a bit brittle. When friends would say, "Oh, I know you'll marry again," Rollene would always brush them off with a summary statement: "Oh, no. Been there, done that."

Imagine my surprise when a lovely young CNN correspondent, Kelly Wallace, suggested I chase down Rollene for an interview. Kelly told me she is Rollene's new daughter-in-law.

Everything about the Rollene Saal I met for coffee—now Mrs. Forma and in her mid-sixties—was soft and subtle. She wore a dash of mauve lipstick and eye shadow, a pink turtleneck, and an antique diamond ring, a gift from her new husband. "It seems so hard-edged now, but I was certain I would never try marriage again," she told me. "I'd been married to a 'bad boy' who never got over being a bachelor. After our divorce, I dated a little. I wasn't looking for Mr. Wonderful, just Mr. Not-So-Bad. But I certainly didn't want to marry Mr. Not-So-Bad."

So what had turned her from a tough-minded business tycoon into a pretty-in-pink wife? She winked, leaned over, touched my hand, and said, "It really is a question of having an open heart. I just married a year ago, and it's amazing how much I like being married! I'm astonished." I couldn't wait to hear the story of what had opened her heart. Again, Rollene leaned forward, a smile curving up one side of her face, like a teenage girl eager to tell her girlfriend about the wonders of her new love.

A mutual friend told Rollene she wanted to introduce her to a man whose wife had passed on and was quite lonely. The friend suggested they have dinner as two couples on a Friday night. Rollene thought it was a nice idea. The following day, her phone rang. A voice said, "Hello? This is Warren."

"Warren who?"

"We're supposed to have dinner Friday night," he said. "I don't think that's a good idea. If we have dinner, two couples, I'll never get to know you. Why don't I pick you up tomorrow morning, and we'll go to my house in the country for the day?"

Rollene thought to herself, "This is a man who knows how to take charge of his life." No sooner had she put down the phone than she called up her daughter and fretted, "What am I doing? I'm going to the country, for the *day,* with a guy I've never met? I'll be trapped!"

"Mom, tomorrow's the anniversary of 9/11," her daughter reminded her. "You'll just be home watching TV all day, recycling that agony."

"You're right."

The next morning, as Warren got out of the car to greet Rollene emerging from her apartment building, he took one look and thought to himself, "I'm going to spend the rest of my life with that woman." He did not tell her that.

They drove out to the country. The weather was cool and misty, so they talked and sat on the bed in his house and watched two of the most romantic movies Rollene had ever seen: *Random Harvest* with Ronald Colman and Greer Garson and *Dodsworth* with Mary Astor and Walter Huston. She found out that Warren had been married twice before and both his wives had died of cancer. She realized, "He only knows happy marriage. His total *modus vivendi,* which he expressed by joking, was 'I don't date. I marry.' "

This spooked Rollene. She couldn't handle all of this warm attention and being made to feel she was the center of his universe. She phoned their mutual friend to warn Warren to back off. But she was intrigued by a man who had such a simple view of the male/female universe. "He was just a very open, easy, loving person with none of the *Sturm und Drang* I was used to. Something in me registered that this was an emotionally available person. I think that's when my heart opened."

So many women in their fifties and sixties are wondering whether or not to take the leap, or at least try to connect with a soulmate. What would the evolved Rollene Saal Forma tell them?

"Now that I've dated and married again, I realize that I could have been married six times! There are so many men out there. They're always coming on the market, and they all want to be married. Who wouldn't want to have a woman to organize your life for you? And now I realize that it's possible to love more than one man in your life. More than two. Maybe even more."

Chapter 25

Sex and the Older Woman

*S*exual pleasure among older married couples who have been together for some time is likely to have far less of the feverish libido-driven urgency it did in earlier phases. For many couples, the metamorphosis from passion to a quieter love is eagerly greeted in the context of their ongoing ease of companionship. They've gained a realistic appreciation of each other's strengths and flaws. Given the emotional security they have achieved together, they worry less about any sudden reverses of affection.

After a speaking engagement at the University of Minnesota, sponsored by no less traditional an entity than the Home Economics Department, I asked if any of the academics and community leaders would like to stay and talk about love, sex, dating, and remarriage among women over 50. Seven stayed, more than eager to talk. One of the women in the Minneapolis group who particularly piqued my interest was a retired journalist in her sixties with silky white hair and a sturdy silhouette encased in a high-necked wool pants suit. She indicated on her questionnaire that she is "passionately enjoying sex with a lover." It turned out that Dorothea was referring to her second husband.

Dorothea told the group that her first marriage, entered into at 19, was turned upside down by the 1960s, when, she recalled with a wink of irony, "The world changed and we were all going to be free souls." Once she became engrossed in the civil rights and antiwar movements, she decided to "liberate" herself from marriage and fully enjoyed being single from age 30 to 35 in the pre-AIDS era. By now, however, Dorothea has been married for thirty years to a man who has clearly become her soul-mate.

"We're enmeshed," she said. "We have breakfast together every morning with people who are involved with us in political and social causes. Then we work out with the same trainer, we even go to the same hairdresser." It sounded as if they were a retired couple, cozy as a pair of comfy old shoes. But no. Her husband is a busy lawyer, a senior partner, and both of them serve on many community boards. The "passionate sex life" she referred to on paper seems to be an extension of the intense commitments they share to social causes and progressive politics. In a follow-up interview, Dorothea was more frank about her sex life: "The difference between sex for men and women as they get older, I think, is that it's an ego thing for men. Women don't keep score. My husband is very affectionate and sex is good, but we often have events at night and we come home and read six newspapers and then just fall asleep."

Dorothea's nightly scenario was familiar to the other women in the group and certainly a common reality for many older couples. But that doesn't mean they're content to give up on sex. Far from it. One of the strongest connectors among older couples continues to be physical intimacy. Almost half of Americans 60 and older are sexually active and intimate at least once a month, according to a survey by the National Council on Aging. That's the good news. A more sobering statistic reveals that of this large population of over-60 men and women who are still enjoying lovemaking, or at least kissing and cuddling, 40 percent of them long for *more* sex.

The greatest obstacle to continuing sexual vitality in the later seasons of life is, of course, the death of a spouse. Only 10 percent of American women between the ages of 55 and 64 are widowed, and 2 percent of men, but 2003 data from the U.S. Census Bureau show a grim escalation of widows after the age of 65—almost 30 percent of women between 65 and 74 have lost a mate; over 50 percent are widowed between the ages of 75 and 84; and over the age of 85, more than three quarters of women are left alone.

Yet many refuse to go celibate into their later years. And for once in their lives, women and men seem to agree about the importance of sex.

Roughly 45 percent of both women and men aged 75 or older agree that sexual activity is a critical part of a good relationship, and about 25 percent of them continue to have sexual relations at least once a week, according to the AARP Sexuality Study. However, a far greater number of women than men over 75 admit they do not particularly enjoy sex at that age (24 percent), or that they would be quite happy if they were never asked to go to bed again (37 percent). Many of the latter women have been widowed and either haven't found a new partner or have been discouraged by the preponderance of older men who are unavailable or who look like emergency room cases waiting to happen.

Notwithstanding, seasoned women remain more optimistic about their present lives and their futures in all age groups after 45. As noted earlier, the MacArthur Foundation studies on aging report that one third of women between 50 and 64 report reaching some major life goal or dream.

The Seasoned Widow

I was delightfully surprised when a widow who sat stiffly through one of my group interviews jotted a note to let me know that she was "enjoying passionate sex with a lover." It was a life choice she did not feel comfortable sharing with people who lived in her conservative city, but she felt strongly that her transformation was one that other widows needed to know was possible.

Alicia had led a sheltered life, married as a virgin and faithful to her husband of many years. She went from her daddy's home to her husband's home and was completely swallowed by his aura. The only tiny part of her life that she could call her own was her board membership on a local historical society. In the vacuum of identity left by her husband's sudden death—illness took him down in a matter of months—she turned back to her interest in the historical society and nurtured that spore of personal value. She found she could make a contribution there, drawing upon her fine arts education. Thus she found herself, in her mid-sixties, at the very beginning of her passage into the Age of Mastery.

Once she made up her mind to create a new life, she progressed with increasing momentum through building a new dream, exploring the romantic passage, and discovering the totally unexpected exhilaration of living in the now. Nothing in her previous life had prepared or permitted her to live this way. Alicia was finally able to break free from the old scripts once she entered the Spontaneous Seventies.

"For me, it takes a lot of courage to try new things," she begins. "I was raised in a very reserved environment where the family rule was 'You do it right the first time.' All my life I've had to struggle with that." As bleak as was the loss of her husband—the man who had defined her world—she had felt a flicker of excitement about the opportunities now open to her. Who was *she,* anyway? Could she try becoming her own person, even make some mistakes, but keep working at it?

"I decided to try to build a new life," she declares, "and the first way was through work." She took a staff job at the historical society and volunteered to raise funds for the local chapter of Habitat for Humanity. "I was eager to know different kinds of people. My husband grew up here, so I lived in his world, which was corporate and interbred and had a very tight social structure."

Alicia found the historical society to be filled with like-minded souls who flaunted their idiosyncrasies; how refreshing! The committed idealists at Habitat were even more exciting new colleagues. She began coming to life again. Starting about six months after her husband's death, Alicia began getting calls from a number of different men, all of whom she had known before, sometimes for decades. "They'd never put out any feelers, but of course, neither did I." She began going out for evenings with them—no physical relationship, just a kiss hello and good night—but they were good companions and very attentive. "They're all divorced or widowed and terribly lonely," she observes. "They don't have much of a support system."

I remind her that she had mentioned a passionate lover.

"The only one who knows he's my lover is you," she says. A faint blush tints her ears pink. "Everyone else thinks we're friends. My children live abroad, so who knows what they think?"

Does it matter? I ask.

"No."

The divorced man she met through Habitat is very different from her husband. He is "a conservationist deeply committed to a new vision of cities," she explains, with an obviously shared sensibility. They had known each other only casually over the years, but they had soon become close through working together on social projects and helping each other with their health issues. Then came a stunning admission: "It was six years after we started dating before this relationship was consummated."

Why so long?

"It took that long to finally give myself this relationship."

It was probably one of the first selfish pleasures Alicia had ever given herself. But she couldn't allow it until she had worked her way through one of the biggest obstacles faced by widows: "I had to believe that nothing I do in my present life can change or dishonor or intrude on the relationship I had with my husband." She also had to uncorset herself from the religious proscriptions with which she had grown up: "My faith doesn't encourage intimacy out of wedlock. But this relationship is such a nurturing, blissful thing, I cannot imagine that the God I believe in would think this is evil."

It was a revelation to her that sex could still be exciting at their age. "I had the stereotype in my mind that sex is not something that old people engage in. I think that's a stereotype all around the world. My sex life with my husband had been satisfying, and he was only sick for a short time before he died. I couldn't sleep for two years afterwards. The lack of intimacy is the most devastating thing about being widowed. And I was menopausal. My osteoporosis was getting worse." As part of the preparation for giving herself the new relationship, she researched hormone replacement therapy and found an endocrinologist who gave her an estrogen implant. It did wonders.

But among the cascade of new experiences that have turned her seventies into one of the most vivid stages in her life, none has been more surprising than her new ability to live in the present.

"It's a struggle for me not to try to structure my future," she admits, "which was always my natural propensity. Even to this day, I don't know if this will ever work into a marriage situation." Alicia is not fretting about it one way or the other. Her work is very demanding, she says, and her lover is a tremendous support to her emotionally. Occasionally, the two will go out for supper together, but most of the time they see each other in one of their homes. "This relationship is still not public," she says, and one gets the distinct impression that that makes it all the more spontaneous.

"I'm pretty determined to live a little"—she exhales with a strong gust of laughter—"it's time!"

Grandlove, then, can range from the affectionate closeness of trusted companionship all the way to the unexpected exuberance of seasoned sex.

The Gift of Grandlove

A tender illustration of the selfless quality of grandlove in a relationship that is shadowed by oncoming dementia is a short story by the Canadian writer Alice Munro, "The Bear Came Over the Mountain," from her collection *Hateship, Friendship, Courtship, Loveship, Marriage*. In it, Grant's wife is 70 years old but still upright and trim. "Her hair, which was as light as milkweed fluff, had gone from pale blond to white somehow without Grant's noticing exactly when, and she still wore it down to her shoulders."

They had slept together just about every night for fifty years. What they loved best were "the five or ten minutes of physical sweetness just after they got into bed—something that did not often end up in sex but reassured them that sex was not over yet."

But the wife has begun wandering off, forgetting how to get home, forgetting how long ago they moved into the house they have occupied for twelve years. When the time comes to take her to the kind of place where few of the elderly go willingly, her husband can think only of the girl she was when she proposed to him and he could feel the teenage lust "flashing along all the nerves of her tender new body."

The home has a rule that new residents are not allowed to be visited for the first month. The husband is tortured by the absence of his soulmate. When he returns, will she be one of the blank-eyed or desperately babbling, busy living alternate lives in their heads? But quite a different transformation awaits him. His wife treats him with polite distraction. She is engrossed in a bridge game. But she isn't even playing. She is sitting close beside her new "friend," a man whom she knew as a young girl.

A few more visits, and Grant realizes that he cannot demand of her that she remember him as her husband of nearly fifty years. She is so utterly taken up with her new friend, and radiant. Then one day, suddenly, she takes to her bed stricken with grief. The wife of her new friend has come to take him back home. Grant's wife stops eating, stops walking, cannot stop weeping. He can see that she is in danger of being banished to the floor where they send the blank-eyed babblers.

He seeks out the other wife, a coarse and somewhat mercenary woman with a "walnut-stain tan," and begs her to return her husband to the rest home. She flatly refuses: too expensive. Whereupon Grant takes it on himself to romance this woman, determined to break her down. In the end, he is determined to bring back to his soulmate the only happiness she can now experience—living together in the rest home with her new lover.

Chapter 26

How to Retire
When You're Still Wired

*W*omen over 60 today belong to the first generation of female professionals who broke into male preserves and anchored their adult identity in their jobs and titles. So it's not surprising that many of them are having withdrawal pangs similar to those that men complain about when they face retirement. Boomers of both sexes refuse to accept conventional notions of retirement. Not for them is commitment to eternal play, rest, and mom-and-pop motor trips. They aren't eager to be shuttled off to the golf course full-time, shorn of the structure, professional relationships, and sense of productive value that once defined them.

Marlene Sanders's Solution

One of the earliest women to gain face time on TV as a network news correspondent was Marlene Sanders. Her television career was launched in 1955, when she assisted Mike Wallace in launching one of the first nightly news broadcasts, *Mike Wallace and the News,* on WABD in New York. Nine years later this good-looking woman with a no-nonsense manner and soothingly low voice had earned her own TV news broadcast on ABC. She remained an on-camera presence until her early sixties, pushing the age barrier for a grateful class of newswomen who were hired in the 1970s once antidiscrimination laws were in force.

Marlene's last TV appearance was in the early 1990s. "I was not young, and I had been doing this since the 1950s," she told me. "The truth is, I was tired of it. And I was dismayed by the deterioration of network news."

Now in her mid-seventies, Marlene has remained a very active broadcast presence by doing voice-overs and narrating documentaries. "I'm a very energetic person," she told me when we met for lunch at a café adjacent to the New York Public Library. That was obvious by her still-striking presence, a ginger-haired woman in a streak of a black pants suit, whose engagement in news and the arts makes her a delightful conversationalist. "But I'm not ambitious in the way I used to be," she said. "What I want to do is keep relevant, use what I know, and have a structure."

Like many energetic professional women around her age, Marlene is definitely not ready to retire, but she doesn't feel like killing herself in a full-time job. The free time she has when she's not recording she uses with relish to take a weekly painting class, go to the gym, and pitch in with her sister activists as a contributor to Women's eNews, a website that disseminates information of particular relevance to women. She keeps up with world events as an elected member of the Council on Foreign Relations and teaches as an adjunct professor at New York University.

The structure of her private life was shaken when her husband of many years, Jerry Toobin, the former manager of NBC's Symphony of the Air and longtime director of public affairs for New York's PBS station, died in 1984. Marlene did a lot of dating in the first ten years following that loss, expecting that she would be remarried at some point. "But as the years went on, I began to realize I was doing fine," she told me. "I'm out every night. I go to the opera with friends. I go to the theater a lot by myself. I go to the Philharmonic. I'm over seventy, and I still date—it's the tonic of life.

"But what do you do when you're widowed or divorced and your formerly full professional life comes to an end?" she asked rhetorically. She has found a peer group in The Transition Network, where everybody else is wrestling with the same question. TTN's goal is to help women transition from a family- and career-centered stage into a new phase of growth and renewal. "Unlike fifty years ago, everybody is still figuring out what to do next. It's nice to have company in sorting it all out."

What Webs Women Weave

Most Americans in their late fifties and sixties want to work less, switching to work that is more flexible, less demanding, and more meaningful. Yet both private- and public-sector employers generally induce, or coerce, many employees into retiring earlier, by forcing them to make an either/or choice: continue to work full-time, year-round, or give up their jobs altogether.

Many cannot afford to give up gainful employment in their late fifties or early sixties, if for no other reason than wanting to help their adult children buy a house or save for the stratospherically escalating cost of the grandkids' college education. During the Nineties, the majority of the American population saw a decrease in their expected retirement income. The decline of traditional defined-benefit pension plans, the inexorable rise of health care costs, and the push by conservatives to persuade employees to accept more privatization of their retirement accounts, subject to the volatility of the stock market, is all part of a reversal of the whole concept of "security" for the later years. While wealthy Americans have benefited from generous tax cuts, middle- and lower-income employees have been saddled with chronic insecurities regarding their "golden years."

Women have one great advantage when faced with the forced transition out of full-time employment: they are incredibly active and imaginative when it comes to creating networks of companionship, fun, and purposeful activity to sustain them. An example of women's adaptation is the Red Hat Society, a group formed in 1998 when five seasoned ladies, inspired by Jenny Joseph's poem "Warning," donned the red hat and purple dress of the poem's protagonist and went out together. "When I am an old woman I shall wear purple / With a red hat which doesn't go, and doesn't suit me." Each member of the group had friends who wanted to join, and before long it became an official society. Today, the group boasts more than a million members, the majority over the age of 50 (members under 50 wear lavender dresses and pink hats), and forty thousand chapters in twenty-six countries.

The main objective of the Red Hat Society is to maintain the spontaneity and fun usually associated with youth. While individual chapters often hold fund-raising events for charities of their choice, the society at large has nothing to do with do-gooding. Instead, it's about squeezing as much enjoyment out of life for oneself and one's "sisters." As the Red Hat Society theme song states quite clearly, "All my life, I've done for you. Now it's my turn to do for me."

The Red Hat Society's success lies in connecting a vast web of women. They organize conventions and trips together. They are also connected through the Red Hat Society official website (www.redhatsociety.com), and weekly postings or e-mails sent out to all members. But the most delightful aspect is the face-to-face contact. If a Red Hatter is traveling and she alerts the society, other Red Hatters—highly identifiable in even the busiest of airports—mass at the gate, ready to sweep their sister off to tea and a grand tour of their home city. If a Red Hatter undergoes terrifying or painful medical treatment, the broadcast alerts the society and the unlucky Hatter is often inundated with visits, flowers, and messages of love and support. Perhaps most significantly, whatever life challenges a Red Hatter is facing, she knows there's at least one other Red Hatter out there somewhere whom she can contact and commiserate with. This immense network allows mid- to late-life women to do what they do best: support one another.

The Transition Network (www.thetransitionnetwork.com) is a more localized example of the power of women's networks. Based in New York City (although it may eventually go national), TTN is a nonprofit with more than eight hundred members, mostly career women in their fifties and sixties, from a wide range of professions. They organize peer groups around specific interests, life stages, or location. There are also special-interest groups, such as book clubs or investment groups, and lectures by top professionals in relevant fields. These gatherings are designed to help women help one another with the often scary choices of their life stage. Whether it be how to retire, how to avoid retirement, how to age healthfully, how to start one's own business, or how to deal with death or divorce, a TTN peer group can provide advice, experience, and, most valuably, empathy.

A more established community of preeminent New York women leaders of diverse achievement is Women's Forum, Inc. Its membership is limited to three hundred women in the professional, artistic, and business worlds who come together to make a difference for one another and take leadership roles in matters of importance to them—a model old-girls' network. At the annual convention of the International Women's Forum, I talked with several members about their solutions to the tricky transition from high-wire work to semiretirement.

Staying Power

Professional women who are younger than their husbands and thus get a later start up the ladder are likely to be working long after their husbands retire and bringing in the heavier share of preretirement income. An illustrious member of the Women's Forum, Bettie Alexander Steiger, talked about how she and her husband of forty-nine years had reached the happiest, most harmonious stage of their relationship from their mid-sixties into their early seventies. But their passage into the Grand-love stage went through several very bumpy years and required a great deal of trial and effort to straighten out.

Early on, Bettie had dropped out of the corporate world to raise her children. Her husband, Don, was a career Army officer, and they were constantly moving. Bettie says she wouldn't give up one of those days with her children. She was confident she would have the wit and skills to make up for lost time when she was ready to jump back on the corporate treadmill, which she did, at 42. "It's because I invented the Steiger Theory of out and up—I would stay with a company only until I realized they weren't going to recognize my ability and promote me, just because I didn't have the 'time and grade,' as they say in the Army. Instead, I'd find another company that would hire me at a higher level." Bettie changed corporate colors six times in the next ten years. "Most women are so afraid to take a chance."

At the age of 52, Bettie was ready to seize a new dream. Her employer, Xerox, saw that she was about ready to leave the company and offered to create an exciting position for her. It sent her from the East Coast out to PARC, its former research center in Palo Alto, California, where she enjoyed a high-testosterone role running the company's technology and innovation group. Bettie worked with the brightest propeller heads coming out of Stanford and other high-tech institutions, hiring hungry MBAs. With them, she focused her marketing skills on commercializing the company's technological research.

I first met Bettie when she joined Women's Forum West, which offered a built-in network of friends and professional contacts. She has a warm and lively alto voice, a staccato mind, and an extroverted personality. She connects easily with new people and knows how to build their egos. Although she is not a notably attractive woman, she carries herself with the confidence of one who knows she is desired. When we got to know each other, she was frank in telling me why.

"Don and I have a wonderful sex life. It's active today, and it's very innovative. He had a triple bypass seven years ago. He's in great shape, but he has a congenital cholesterol problem. He's still able to perform sex, but he doesn't feel like it as strongly as he would like to. So this is something we talk about. He is still able to gratify me in other ways, and I have discovered that I can satisfy him by being patient."

Bettie told me one of her secrets. Her husband is an early riser. Bettie comes up for breakfast about two hours later, but she never leaves the bedroom without doing her stretches and putting on her makeup. "I come upstairs looking great. One of the things that I think keeps me wanting to be attractive is him. He'll tell me, 'You're beautiful.' I always thought I was ugly. But I don't feel that anymore. I told him it's because he still desires me."

The Steigers had put the Sexual Diamond idea into practice. "We had a deal," says Bettie. "If I got a chance to move up the ladder and it required us to move, he would move for my career. I'd already moved for his career nineteen times." Don kept his promise and left behind all his structure and his friends at the Pentagon. There was no ready social infrastructure in their new California home. Not long after the move, Bettie had to sit Don down and say, "We have to talk about this. Your image in your life is diminishing. You've got to get involved." Don began taking an interest in their home owner's association, managing their finances, and eventually took over management of a wheat ranch.

But there was a period when they had too much time together, Bettie says. When her company offered her an attractive buyout, she decided to try retirement. "We were faced with each other all the time—it was the worst time in our married life."

Bettie realized she was definitely not cut out for kicking back. She started her own company, Steiger Associates, to consult with start-up companies on business strategies. She is now 71 and just starting another new business. "Don has learned to understand that I need to have absolute independence in making decisions about what I want to do and where I want to go. That has been a transition in his thinking, because he was an Army man used to hierarchy." The beauty of having her own business is that she can dictate when she will take a vacation. Like most older couples, Bettie and Don find that a vacation always stimulates their relationship. They go to Hawaii for four weeks of the year and hope someday to ramp it up to two months of the year.

"My being successful in the late part of our life has really helped our financial situation," Bettie says. "Don's ego is not diminished by my success. It never was. He's always taken great pride in what I do. This is the mellowest and most fun time in our marriage, because we finally understand and accept each other."

How Long Do You Plan to Live?

But there won't be much that is mellow or fun about the retirement years if you are not healthy. When I ask my interviewees, "How long do you plan to live?," the most common answers are "As long as I'm healthy enough to enjoy it," "As long as I can take care of myself," and "As long as my mind is clear."

The problem is, by the time we reach our mid-sixties, give or take, we don't get those choices. Given the rapid pace of medical technology, most of us will live longer than we expected—whether we like it or not. We've all heard too many hard-living celebrities lament, in the misery of their later years, "If only I'd known how long I would live, I would have taken better care of my body."

We now know that after our mid-fifties, when most women are past menopause, 70 percent of aging is controlled by our lifestyle: how actively we move around, how much we drink or smoke, how well we sleep, how many close friends we keep up with, and how engaged we remain in life and community.

Even more impressive is a newer scientific estimate: half of all of the sickness and serious accidents we are told to anticipate after we turn 50 can be virtually eliminated, if we learn how to live younger.

Wouldn't you like to be able to hike a mountain in your seventies? Dance in your eighties? Entertain in your own condo in your nineties? And continue to enjoy sexual intimacy, skin to skin, from 45 to death?

My friends have always teased me about being an exercise nut. What's even weirder is the fact that I *enjoy* exercise—especially when I feel the strings of my muscles tighten and those delicious endorphins washing the bad mood out of my brain. Now comes new information from biologists that most of the cells in our bodies are designed to disintegrate after brief life spans. Our blood cells are replaced every three months. Our muscles are new every four months. And our bones dissolve and rebuild every couple of years. This programmed decay is thought to be nature's way of allowing us to adapt to changing living conditions, and to counteract the fact that older cells tend to be less resistant to contaminants.

The object of daily exercise is to live long, die short. That isn't as simplistic a slogan as it sounds.

The concept is supported by scientific studies of body and brain chemistry. It's all spelled out by Henry S. Lodge, M.D., and Chris Crowley, authors of a new book titled *Younger Next Year for Women: Live Like You're 50—Strong, Fit, Sexy—Until You're 80 and Beyond,* being published concurrently with this book. Dr. Lodge, an internist and gerontologist at the Columbia Medical School, clearly describes the seesaw of growth and decay.

Basically, the idea is this: Exercise is the master signaler that triggers the cycles of strengthening and repair within your muscles and joints. To signal the cells of your body to grow anew, then, you must work your muscles. Exercise also contributes to positive chemical changes in the brain. Daily exercise, claims Dr. Lodge, leads directly to younger life, with its heightened immune system, better sleep, and resistance to heart attacks, stroke, hypertension, arthritis, and Alzheimer's disease. It also leads to improved sexuality. "But let your muscles sit idle," he cautions, "and decay takes over again."

Sure, you can sit back and start resting at 70—you deserve it, right?— and rest your way all the way to the rest home. Or you can start now, growing your body new a little bit every day, and avoiding decay. Dr. Lodge says we have to commit to exercising six days a week until they carry us off into the sunset. That's right, six days. Four of them need to be serious aerobic exercise. Two of the others need to build in strength training. You may not want to hear this advice, but you know it's true. Some need it more than others.

Kids, you know who you are.

Menopause gets blamed for lots of unpleasant changes that often catch women by surprise after 50: Gaining weight. Losing energy. Arthritic pains and muscle aches. We hate having the excuse taken away, but the scientific facts are what they are. Women gain weight faster after 50 because our metabolism slows down, and the only way to combat that aging effect is by eating less and exercising more. *In every decade of our life we move roughly 10 percent less.* The more sedentary we are, the less energy we have. And the aches and pains of aging are exaggerated when our muscles are allowed to go slack and our joints are not stretched and lubricated on a regular basis.

Up until menopause, decay is slower in women than in men. But peri-menopause jump-starts the decay process, and for the duration of the transition it's like being on a runaway snow saucer, spinning downhill over the bumps of accelerated bone loss, oncoming arthritis, and diminishing defenses against heart disease, cancer, and depression. The chemical that induces the decay process through inflammation is counteracted by a chemical known as C-10 that produces repair and growth. All forms of aerobic exercise stimulate the C-10 growth chemical in both the muscle cells and the bloodstream. When we are sedentary, although we won't feel it, the body's muscles and organs are receiving a slow, steady drip of inflammation. When we do enough aerobic exercise to sweat for at least twenty minutes, we set off a torrent of blood coursing through the muscles to the heart, bones, organs, and brain, carrying the rejuvenating bath of C-10 growth-and-repair chemical.

The kind of aerobic exercise I'm talking about is age-appropriate and effective, and does not mean killing yourself running 10K or hiking Mount Kilimanjaro. We're talking about biking, swimming, speed-walking, cross-country skiing, and rowing—the healing sports. You can also hit the mark by going to the gym and using the treadmill, the elliptical machine, or the stationary rowing machine. Unfortunately, the kind of aerobic activity that is going to prolong your life does not include tennis doubles or golf. They are both delightful sports for your muscles and your attitude, but they are not aerobic. Singles tennis is fine, so long as you pant, but a tennis pro once told me that during an hour's worth of a doubles match, the ball is actually in play for only four and a half minutes. And sadly, nobody ever got a bath of C-10 from riding around in a golf cart.

So, if we are disciplined about doing some form of serious aerobic exercise four days a week, and strength training two of the other days, the gerontologist warrants that we will reduce the risk of breast cancer by as much as 50 percent, and have a sporting chance of being able to dance our feet off at age 80.

Discovering a New Dream Every Bonus Decade

I am privileged to count as a friend and life coach the co-founder of Rancho la Puerta, Deborah Szekely. A true pioneer who helped give birth to the fitness revolution, she has committed her life to living naturally in an increasingly artificial world. One of her secrets is to invent a new dream for every one of the bonus decades after 60.

"I really believe that I am who I am because, when I turned sixty, I made a radical change," she says. She loved the ranch and her other creation, the Golden Door; she loved the staff and just about everything she did. "But I'd been doing it long enough, since I was eighteen." Deborah left the business in the care of her son, Alex, and moved to Washington, where she found a new dream as head of a government agency. She found that hands-on management skills were not only transferable to government bureaucracy, but equally valid in the nonprofit organizations of Latin America and the Caribbean. Six years later, having changed the way that much of grassroots development there was carried out, Deborah was restless again.

"I'm looking for something to lose sleep over again," she told everyone.

She found it by launching her own nonprofit agency, which was dedicated to finding and training inner-city leaders. She was in perpetual motion for the next decade, flying among four different cities to supervise her program. When she had time to drop into the ranch, she would tell guests, "Every time you change careers, every time you make a move, it gets all of your adrenaline flowing, it renews your energy." And she was living proof.

In her late seventies, she came back to the ranch to help her son, who was stricken with melanoma. Deborah refreshed her old dream by finding and introducing newer healing arts, such as Pilates, Feldenkrais, and NIA. She also developed a technique for cleansing her days of useless "shoulds" and boring people.

"Look back at your calendar for the last week," she advises her guests. "We're all so busy planning for tomorrow and next week, but you can learn a lot by looking at how you spent the last week." She advises getting out colored pencils and underlining in a different color the ways you spent your time: How am I treating myself? Did I have a lot of fun? Did I learn anything? What do I have to show for last week? And what did I do that was a total waste of time?

In 2005 Deborah advanced to the age of 83. She had buried her son, grieved, and launched a new concept for the ranch—women's weeks in the off-season of August, which attracted many newcomers to the ranch, notably women whose inner image is "too old" or "too fat" and who've never felt comfortable in skimpy workout togs when men are around. It was a big hit. Deborah herself still hikes the mountain at the ranch. "I'd be embarrassed in front of my guests *not* to do it. That doesn't mean I'm going for the top, as I used to on my good days, but it does mean I can do a really good hourlong hike." Deborah anticipates that she probably has another twenty years on her life's journey. And once more she's restless. Time for a new dream. What she has found to lose sleep over again is founding and chairing the New Americans Immigration Museum and Learning Center.

Chapter 27

Seasoned Sirens

*W*ho would ever have imagined that the love story that would captivate the world in 2005 would feature a divorcée with a doughy body and weathered countenance who had waited 58 years for her prince to come? To believe it, one only had to see the wraparound smile of Camilla Parker-Bowles as she returned the love shining in the eyes of Prince Charles. By now, he was a balding gent given to making high-minded speeches and ducking the disapproving gaze of his dour mother, the queen of England, who once referred to Camilla as being "rather used."

It turns out that being "rather used" is one of Camilla's more seductive qualities. Years of being battered by life and sustaining her love through scandal, revilement by Diana supporters, and ridicule by the pitiless British press had tested the love and loyalty of the prince's paramour. All those years of hide-and-seek *liaisons dangereuses,* while Princess Diana was alive and during her virtual sainthood following her tragic death, probably only intensified Camilla's allure in the eyes of the tightly corseted prince.

Camilla combines the full mammary comfort of maternal warmth with the spanking baritone of a British nanny. Yet the promise in her eyes, and in her party décolleté, is that of uninhibited ravishment, a role for which she was primed by her great-grandmother, Alice Keppel, the adulterous lover of King Edward VII. In her fifties, Camilla can clomp around in the unglamour of tweeds because she's comfortable with who she is. Possessed of the wisdom accumulated through close contact with the practice of statecraft, she has become her husband's most intimate adviser. The two have obviously become as comfortable with each other as a pair of well-worn Wellingtons. You can sense in them what I mean by the quiet joy of Grandlove.

It bears repeating: Women's lives are long and have many seasons. Seductresses in their later years have always been able to cast a great spell over both men and women. Their enchantments combine a fully enriched character, a sharp mind, endlessly rechargeable vitality, status, glamour, and a contagious spirit. They operate on dual current, able to switch back and forth between maternal warmth and high-voltage sexuality. I call such women seasoned sirens.

Oprah and Tina

Among the contemporary pantheon of seasoned American sirens, the star of stars has to be Oprah Winfrey. Since she entered her fifties, she has worn her hair long and curly; her face, by whatever secret means, looks more beautiful than ever; and she has settled into the sleeker but still bumptious silhouette that her body seems meant to inhabit. She exudes the confident spontaneity of the accomplished senior siren.

Like many older seductresses, Oprah apparently sees no need to marry. She has her own empire and a low-maintenance, live-out escort in Steadman. That leaves her free to flirt overtly with much younger heartthrobs like the Academy Award–winning actor Jamie Foxx, who declared his love for her on the *Oprah* show. And she seems proud to shake her booty in public appearances, as noted by Tina Brown in her newspaper column commenting on the *grandes dames* honored by New York Women in Communications at its 2005 Matrix awards luncheon at the Waldorf-Astoria. "There was something so glorious about the confident roll of Oprah's behind in its tight couture suit as she powered up to the podium to present an award . . ."

We build on the boldness of the seasoned sisters who go before us. Oprah wasn't looking forward to midlife. But in an interview with Tina Turner for her own magazine, America's mother confessor made an admission of her own. "It was because of you that I decided to rock on through the fifties," she told Tina Turner. "It was because of you that I said, 'I'm not going to stay where I am. I'm going to get better.' " Following her resolution, Oprah has not only expanded the reach of her TV show to 111 countries, she continues to offer inspirational ideas in *O: The Oprah Magazine,* which marked its fifth-anniversary issue in 2005. She also finds new channels all the time to invest her fame in social action.

And who wouldn't be inspired by Tina Turner, a senior siren now past 65 and still stunning? The survivor of a brutal marriage who busted out of it with thirty-six cents in her pocket, she went on to shatter the age ceiling as an international rock and soul legend whose sexy concerts were among the top sellers in history. She has spent her middle years living contentedly in Zurich with a lover sixteen years her junior.

Anna the Vamp of Tarzana

Anna Boyce knows something about how to grow old and keep her groove. She is not famous, except among her former constituents in Orange County, where she is a retired assemblywoman and congresswoman. She is a 74-year-old contemporary California gal, tiny, twice widowed, sassy-tongued, with spiky carrot-colored hair and mischievous eyes. She likes to keep two or three men on the string at all times—at least one of them younger.

"Younger men are a lot more energetic," she told the members of WomanSage in our group interview, "and they don't try to pull that Viagra trick like the older men do."

It was on her third dinner date with an older man, and she had gone to the ladies' room. When she returned, there was a blue pill sitting on her dessert plate. "What's that for?" she asked. "That's our dessert," he said.

"Obviously, he did not come home with me," she says in high dudgeon.

I call her Anna the Vamp of Tarzana. It's a title she has earned after being widowed and alone for more than eight years, having dated more than her fair share of widowers, and having worked out a foolproof barrier against their horny persuasions. "Right off the bat I tell them I'm not available sexually unless there's chemistry," she tells us. "Usually after four or five dates, the pressure starts. First I tell them it can't be in my house—I only have a single bed. The truth is, I'm not going to be the one who gets up and leaves in the middle of the night. Then I say I want a blood test done. They always swear they haven't been with anyone else for years, I'm the first. I say, fine, but I require a blood test, and I'll have one too, and that will set the stage. Nobody has brought me a blood test yet, not one man."

She pauses. "Am I blushing?"

We want to know if she enjoyed sex when she was married. Oh yes, she says, very much. And she misses it. But she finds that when she takes the pressure off older men to perform sexually, they're relieved, and they keep coming back for the next date. "I haven't lost any of the ones I like," she says, letting her lashes flutter demurely. "They're mainly looking for the same things women are at this age—companionship, friendship, oh, and someone to listen to the stories of their past. I've heard so many war stories, I feel like I was right in the trenches with them in World War II!"

What she enjoys most about dating is the flirting, the game. "It's a challenge to keep them interested in you—I like that part," she says, adding with a slightly avaricious giggle, "and the little gifts—the perfume and jewelry and theater—being picked up and taken to really nice places, having that male attention all around you—it's definitely not like being with my children and grandchildren."

History's Seasoned Sirens

Throughout history, seasoned sirens have enjoyed the dangerous liberty of postmenopausal freedom, allowing them to escape domesticity and flirt and flit among male admirers, or to become the intimate advisers of powerful men. In her delightful book *Seductress,* the historian Betsy Prioleau points out that some of the most celebrated senior goddesses throughout history were not beautiful. In fact, some were downright homely, but their other charms nonetheless captivated powerful men and creative geniuses, and they often became the most intimate advisers to kings and princes of Europe, presidents and statesmen.

For men, she observes, the older woman is always "mother," "a source of terrifying dependencies, authority, and incest taboos. Also, of course, a source of tremendous appeal. The cagey Silver Foxes handled this high-intensity aphrodisiac with finesse, artfully mixing nurturer and sex queen so as to neutralize oedipal anxieties and maximize maternal hit." And as these historical seductresses grew older, they were even more delightfully spontaneous, with what Prioleau dubs a "what-the-hell closing time joie de vivre."

Diane de Poitiers

A dominant seasoned siren in sixteenth-century France was Diane de Poitiers (1499–1566). Her mentor was one of Europe's boldest iconoclasts, Anne de Beaujeu, who provided the 15-year-old Diane with a rich husband forty years her senior, calculating that he would bestow upon the girl the benefits of early widowhood. When he obliged by dying, Diane assumed the role for which she had been groomed, chatelaine of their estate in Burgundy. Now, along with the charms of the seasoned siren and maternal tutor, she had the additional benefits of wealth and status. The 17-year-old Henri, future king of France, fell madly in love with her. As Prioleau notes, "she initiated the future king sexually when he was only seventeen and ruined him for other women."

Under the guidance of Diane de Poitiers, the prince emerged from his awkward adolescence, read widely, and enjoyed festivities organized by his paramour. Prioleau paints a vivid picture: "Henri played the guitar with Diane in his lap, stopped to fondle her breasts, and turned to the company and asked if they'd ever seen a more beautiful woman."

Her beauty was only in the eyes of her besotted beholder. To any objective eye, Diane was downright homely, with a poker face, narrow lips, and no eyelashes. But like all seasoned sirens, she practiced futuristic anti-aging regimes that made her more appealing. For a sixteenth-century European woman, she was uniquely pleasant to kiss, because she cleaned her teeth with a vinegar-soaked rag. She bathed daily in ice-cold water, and her complexion remained clear of smallpox scars, another rarity for a woman of her time. She also rode horseback and kept her slim, lithe figure into her forties, when she appeared at least two decades younger.

It wasn't only her tight riding costumes and décolleté gowns that kept the king intrigued; she also became a mistress of statecraft. The king admitted her to his private counsel, an unprecedented position for a woman in French history, and, as his chief adviser, she forged alliances and negotiated peace treaties. Her enduring credo is worth remembering for all those who aspire to be seasoned sirens.

"You must dazzle."

Minette Helvetius

Benjamin Franklin also preferred older to younger women, even when he was the most recognized and admired American of the late eighteenth century. When Franklin was sent to Paris in 1776 to secure French aid for the Revolution, he was a high-spirited 70-year-old who represented the new world's self-made man. He immediately became the darling of the radical chic set, pursued by young Parisian lovelies. Yet his heart was captured by a widow in her sixties.

Minette Helvetius had re-created herself upon the death of her husband in 1771. She'd bought a cozy house in the Paris suburb of Auteuil, where, once a week, with shrieks of joy and a flourish of her short, girlish petticoats, she greeted the intellectual and political elite at her coveted salon. They were mostly men, of course, a coterie she entertained with comic anecdotes and led through the night in rowdy drinking songs.

Minette seduced Franklin with her powers of rejuvenation. Around her, the portly septuagenarian confessed, he felt "like a little boy." So enamored did the famous American inventor and diplomat become of this shameless seasoned siren, he told friends that he intended to "capture her and keep her with him for life." According to Prioleau's research, Minette also fell very much in love with Franklin, but she steadfastly refused to marry him, remaining devoted to her salon and her personal freedom. She and Franklin, though, remained ardent lovers, exchanging letters and regular visits, kissing in public, and praising each other on both sides of the Atlantic.

Again, this seasoned French siren seemed to age backward. She awoke early, ran about her estate with the caretaker's children, and continued to draw a circle of admirers until she died, at the astonishing age—for an eighteenth-century woman—of 81.

Today's Senior Goddesses

The seasoned sirens of today don't have to seduce men to hang on to their position. A track record of being witty, whip-smart, superambitious, high-energy performers in whatever career field they choose allows them to take control of their own lives. And that counts far more in the long run toward attaining the rank of seasoned siren than being a young blond airhead whose outer charms will fade and eventually reveal a vacuousness underneath.

Perhaps the most visible group of seasoned sirens in the public eye today are TV newswomen. After Barbara Walters broke the age barrier, a boomlet of ambitious women journalists have soared to top-visibility positions and are continuing to hold those coveted on-camera spots into their sixties—another evidence of the tectonic change in attitudes toward seasoned women. Mavericks, they all broke rank with the codes of pre-feminist behavior, ran with their ambitions, seized male privilege, and defied convention. They had their children late or not at all. They worked twice as hard as their male counterparts. The smartest ones married men who proudly championed, and in some cases fostered, their big careers; or they didn't marry or remarry but kept on trucking. And they all know how to tell a great story.

That last is a key component of the seasoned siren's charm. Remember Natalie, the South African woman who flourished after her husband left her in Santa Fe? She makes it her business to pick up enough knowledge, by reading and interacting with all kinds of people, so she can keep up a lively conversation with any one of the hundred-plus people who are invited to her New Year's Eve party. It was the French novelist and essayist André Maurois who wrote, "A happy marriage is a long conversation which always seems too short."

Breakfast TV viewers are drawn to *Good Morning America*'s co-host Diane Sawyer, who isn't new or different, but eternally smooth and compassionate. Diane has maintained the same radiant golden girl looks and crackling intelligence that allowed her to break into broadcasting in 1967. Whether she is delivering the news of the day or bantering with her male co-host, Charles Gibson, she always keeps the buzz going between sexual allure and confident authority.

It's interesting to step back and recall the prognostications some of today's senior goddesses made more than a decade ago about how long they thought they could last as women on camera in a field where the bosses are still men.

Lesley Stahl, who joined the exclusive club of millionaire news stars in her mid-forties, broke into the TV business with "the class of '72," when affirmative action demonstrated that broadcasting was rife with sexism. Lesley was hired by CBS News as a Washington-based reporter. Like the rest of the early TV seductresses, she was not only a beauty, she was a smart workaholic, willing to get up in the middle of the night to go to work and keep a suitcase packed for departure at a moment's notice. She didn't marry until her mid-thirties, to a handsome younger writer, Aaron Latham, and she didn't give birth to her only child, Taylor Latham, until her late thirties. She made these choices in favor of a solid personal life while believing—erroneously as it turns out—they would limit her career. In 1988, she told Marlene Sanders for her book *Waiting for Prime Time,* "I cannot go after things like *60 Minutes* because I have a child and it would be a sacrifice, but I have my child and it's wonderful, it's my life."

Voilà! In 1991, Lesley Stahl was plucked from her estimable position as anchor of CBS's *Face the Nation* to be the sole female anchor of *60 Minutes,* following Diane Sawyer. Lesley has maintained her position on camera at *60 Minutes* for more than fifteen years, seemingly ageless, still attractive as a woman, and more appealing than ever as an interpreter of cultural trends.

This makes my point once more: women's lives are long and have many seasons.

The number of older stars still burning in the galaxy of TV newswomen grows each year. Andrea Mitchell has held her high post as NBC's chief foreign affairs correspondent for a number of years. Cokie Roberts remains the senior news analyst for NPR and the trusted political commentator for ABC News, as well as having become a best-selling author. Lynn Sherr is continuing well into her sixties as a high-profile news and feature reporter at ABC News. Betty Rollin, another attractive veteran in her sixties, offers special reports on the *NBC Nightly News,* in addition to her prolific record as the author of six books, most memorably *First,*

You Cry, about her successful battle with breast cancer thirty-one years ago. Mary Alice Williams has not only been an anchor on CNN, and formerly vice president in charge of CNN's New York bureau—the second largest in the world—she has done it all in spite of, rather than because of, her extraordinary good looks.

Betsey Aaron, an intrepid foreign correspondent with a track record of dangerous, overseas assignments, had a hunch that women with guts and groundbreaking reporting behind them would have a better chance of surviving their middle age in front of the camera. She has been proven right. Candy Crowley, for instance, CNN's veteran Washington political correspondent, and Lisa Myers, NBC's senior investigative correspondent, are both solid, full-figured fixtures on camera, with great sources and tempered insights. The fact that they look less like models than the middle-aged woman next door only adds to the comfort level of many viewers.

Kitty Carlisle Hart

I couldn't wait to interview one of America's grandest living seasoned sirens. But I had to wait to see her until she returned from Palm Beach, where she was being paid $20,000 to get up on a table every night and sing.

Kitty Carlisle Hart is a hit at 95.

She is arguably the only woman of her age still being booked to sing at supper clubs. Kitty made her New York City nightclub debut on her ninety-fourth birthday. Performing at Feinstein's club at the Regency Hotel on Park Avenue, she sold out all three nights. It jump-started her career all over again, after fifty years, and she is now in great demand around the country.

This is a woman who has spanned almost a century of performing, first, as a clever child who learned to tell diverting stories to assuage her mother's rages, then, in her salad days, by singing in Paris and London in the 1920s as part of her mother's plan to land her "safely in the arms of wealth and suitability." Her early story sounds like that of the ill-fated heroine of Edith Wharton's famous novel *The House of Mirth.* But unlike Lily Bart, who died in the bloom of life, Kitty's full powers as an enchantress of men, a successful entertainer, a legendary culture czar, and a major money draw at cultural benefits did not begin to mature until her early fifties.

In her First Adulthood, Kitty's singing and acting career never quite made it out of the second tier, although she did appear with the Marx brothers in the movie *A Night at the Opera.* She was not a natural beauty. But she was persistent. During her fifteen years of marriage to Moss Hart, the brilliant but manic-depressive playwright, he dressed her in long velvet gowns and helped to shape a new persona; Mrs. Hart played her part as the adoring wife and glamorous socialite who kept them hobnobbing with the cultural royalty of the day. She was 51 when her husband died. "Moss was everything to me," she says. But it's been in the last nearly half century of life on her own that Kitty has put out more vivid blooms, year after year, like a hothouse orchid.

Before entering her East Side Manhattan apartment for our interview, I am told by the elevator man that she came home from the hospital only two days before. "But she's out walking every day, she's amazing."

Normally one to make a dramatic entrance, Mrs. Hart this afternoon wears no makeup whatsoever. Her silver-threaded dark hair is bed-rest tousled. But moments into our conversation, her indefatigable élan kicks in when I pose the first question.

"I'm writing about women who have survived loss, learned how to live alone, created new dreams for themselves, and manage to maintain their magnetism for men and women, no matter what age they are. How do you do it?"

A smile cracks open the eggshell of her face and spreads. "I twinkle."

I ask her what older men need.

"The same thing younger men need. The same thing all men need— somebody to listen to them. And I'm a very good listener."

She has mastered the art of capturing men's hearts, and she has enticed many more than her share of the dashing men of five eras. "I knew George and Ira and Cole and Dick and Irving," she can say in one mouthful, referring to the Gershwin brothers, Cole Porter, Richard Rodgers, and Irving Berlin. George Gershwin proposed to her, "but he never loved me—he just thought me suitable." Sinclair Lewis, the conscience of America in the 1920s and the first American to win the Nobel Prize in Literature, also wanted to marry Kitty. But when he declared he was going to tell his wife, the viciously witty writer Dorothy Thompson, "it scared me to death." In the 1930s, Kitty was swept off her feet by a Brazilian lady-killer, Decio de Moura, who wore a monacle and danced like Valentino, but she left him virtually at the altar in Rio. All the while, Kitty had her eye on a gifted and socially prominent playwright, Moss Hart, who was the "toast of Broadway," as the collaborator with George S. Kaufman on plays such as *You Can't Take It with You, The Man Who Came to Dinner,* and later as a director of *My Fair Lady* and *Camelot.*

Try as she might, she couldn't get the attention of the only man she wanted to marry. "I waited nine years for Moss!" she exclaims. They crossed paths at parties, but Hart never even looked at her. Still single in her mid-thirties, she recalls mourning to her mother, "I'm not married. I don't have any children. I'm going to wind up like Sophie Tucker singing 'Some of These Days' in a café in Montana."

How did she finally capture Moss Hart's attention?

"It was at a party at Lillian Hellman's," she begins, delighted to spin one of the stories she has polished over the years. "Moss was on the arm of the sofa. I wanted him to really look at me. So I said, 'Moss, tell me about your trip to the South Pacific.' " She listened with the rapt attention and expressive responses that seasoned sirens know how to give back, "and he looked at me for the first time." He finally called the next day to ask her out. "He said, 'Are you surprised?' And I said, 'No, I knew you would call.' " Not long after, they became inseparable.

Secrets of Seduction

Kitty added another charm to her arsenal when she had to tame her husband's artistic torments. "I tell a good story. And I'm very amusing." Her husband was a famous insomniac. "We slept in a double bed, and he wouldn't even let me leave the bed to go into the children when they were sick," she said. "He would say, 'Tell me the story of your life again.' " Like Scheherazade, she talked until she'd lulled him to sleep.

"Did that suggest to you that seduction is mainly a head trip?" I ask.

"Yes, I think so." She thinks for a moment. "Now, I don't know about the very young girls who have big bosoms. But to me, the real sex appeal is in the imagination."

It took her some years to overcome her inhibitions in telling stories in a social situation. After one of the Harts' early dinner parties, Kitty bemoaned the fact that she had sat, mummified, while their illustrious guests vied for who could tell the best story. Her husband gave her the secret: "Don't expect every head to turn and people to say, 'Now, Kitty?' You have to *push* your way in." She once found Moss Hart practicing his monologues in the mirror before parties, and she followed suit. When she gave too many details, her husband schooled her, "Don't give us the southern road show version, make it short and punchy."

Appearances are very important to Kitty Hart, as they are to all seasoned sirens. "Discipline is the key," she says. "You never give in to getting old." She practices her own anti-aging techniques. "I lie on the floor and put my legs over my head and touch the ground behind me ten times—don't try it if you haven't been doing it. Then I do thirty leg lifts. I use a treadmill, and I take a walk every day." She also makes it a daily discipline to play scales on the piano. To show the results, she holds out her long, graceful hands with their beautifully straight fingers, the nails manicured bright red.

And what does she do for mental stimulation? She reads a couple of newspapers every day, but she doesn't have time to read books. Why? asks the bruised author in me.

"I'm out every night," she trills. "I spend maybe one night a week at home in three months. I *like* going out. Dinners, parties, charity benefits, theater. I have a box at the opera—one of my beaus loves the opera. And I offer them little dinners, tête-à-tête, at home."

Does she cook? A shrug of utter disdain passes over her face. "I'm not domestic. I am a performer."

The next obvious question is, why, after Moss Hart died, did she never remarry?

"I loved my independence and freedom," she says without hesitation. And she has continued to take full advantage of her independence to keep beaus flattering and fluttering around her over the forty-plus years of her widowhood. Has that been important to maintaining her vitality? I ask.

"Why not? I have three beaus now."

Her youngest heartthrob is 89. Another is now 102; she refers to him as Mr. Neuberger. "He had a big brokerage firm, and they tell me he's very rich." (He is a renowned investor, Roy Neuberger, who founded the firm Neuberger Berman in 1939 to manage money for wealthy individuals; in 2003, it became part of Lehman Brothers.) But it's not money that turns her on. It's knowing that her zest for life and love can keep audiences at her feet. And that she can keep a man in a wheelchair up and singing show tunes with her in a nightclub until the wee hours, to celebrate his 102nd birthday.

Of course, the life of Kitty Carlisle Hart is an orbit away from the lives of most of us, but I offer her story for the sheer inspiration of her life—the long-legged lady with the wreath of dark hair who is still out there, still working, still dazzling, still dangling beaus in her mid-nineties, and looking years younger than many in her audiences who are twenty years her junior.

Chapter 28

Love in the Fourth Dimension

*T*he last thing Donna Brower wanted to do was work with seniors—not when she was 45 and already squirming to escape her own aging process. But there she was, assigned for her social work internship to the Senior Center in Scottsdale, Arizona.

The first time she went to check on the Thursday-afternoon dance session, she was blown away. This was no collection of the halt and lame pushing each other around a linoleum-floored cafeteria. These were women from age 50 to past 100, all wearing high-heeled dance shoes and fluttery skirts, who grabbed their male partners and swung onto the polished wooden dance floor the moment the live music started. They pumped their knees in a fast jitterbug and changed partners to swan about in a slow Viennese waltz and changed again, when the whistle blew, to jostle for the men who excel at slow dancing, men who can hide their Parkinsonian tremors by pressing the women close to their chests.

Suddenly, Donna felt a pinch on her rear end. She marched out to the receptionist with a stricken look on her face. "I'm absolutely shocked!" she said. "One of the gentlemen just goosed me."

Blasé, the receptionist replied, "Get over it, honey. Sex is the last to go."

The Dancing Dolls of Scottsdale

If younger people lump all those over 70 into one indistinguishable, irrelevant, and invisible pool, it's because they haven't been exposed to contemporary senior centers in the dance capital of America. Every winter, thousands of women and men in their fully seasoned years abandon the shut-in months in the northern states to converge on Phoenix and its environs. They come for the same reason, best expressed by one of the regulars at the Thursday dances, Essie Brown, who was interviewed at Scottsdale Senior Center on her 106th birthday. She had outlived three husbands, but she had always found a new dance partner. On this birthday she was looking for another new one because her last partner had just died.

"Does he have to be good-looking?" the interviewer asked.

"No, honey, he just has to know how to move his feet."

"Why do you love to dance?"

"Because it keeps me alive."

And indeed, she stayed alive to the age of 108.

"We run a high school for seniors," jokes Tim Miluk, who manages the center. "Our seniors have the same issues as teenagers: driving, dating, and sex." They don't admit to being "seniors," even if they're in their eighties, and they resent the authorities worrying about whether or not they can drive home safely. They seldom talk openly about sex, referring to a special friend as "my dance partner." But Donna has no doubt that they often pair off after the dances. "There have been a few times where people in the parking lots were seen doing the horizontal mambo." She laughs tolerantly. (After being goosed at the Thursday dance, she has stayed on for a decade as the social services coordinator, and is enlivened by the spirit of these aging live wires.) Invariably, the men say they never liked dancing before, and only in their twilight years do they come to understand what women really want: "Women want to go dancing!"

The men who take the trouble to learn are in overheated demand, since there are six women to every man who frequents the center, most of whom are single. Dee Williams, who runs another dance club in Mesa, says the attendees are the movers and shakers of their age group. "We don't want to just sit around and watch TV, we want to be up and active.

You figure three hours of ballroom dancing is equal to running well over ten miles, and I do it six or seven times a week."

Born in Ohio hillbilly country, Dee was a maverick who escaped early and became a TV producer and later hosted a family show about active older people. When her husband died on Thanksgiving Eve of 1986, she worked out her grief by going to 187 dances the following year. By her late sixties, having lived through too many dark Michigan winters, she sold her house, pocketed her savings, and moved to Mesa, which has sunshine just about eternally. She began frequenting the ballrooms in the desert.

By the calendar, Dee is 72. According to her doctor, her body is about 29. A woman with beautifully stark silver hair and a broad laugh, she is petite and wears what appear to be dainty, open-toed dance shoes. No one would guess that she was born with abnormally tiny and painfully arched feet. A doctor told her she would be in a wheelchair by 50. She rejected the pressure to have surgery and overcame the pain with acupuncture, massage, and belief in her new dream—to be a great dancer. Her ballroom shoes are in fact fortified with steel supports. "I dance almost every dance," she says proudly.

At one of the big ballrooms, she met a new dance partner. They moved well together and found easy pleasure in each other's company. Dee told him she was planning to take a trip around the world. "I want to waltz on the Great Wall of China."

He asked if she was going alone. She said yes. He said he'd like to accompany her.

"So we partnered up and we did it together," she says, "like brother and sister. We got two beds. You can do that when you're past the age of nesting. You become people again—male, female, it doesn't make any difference. It's true for a lot of the men too; because the pressure is off of them, they can be themselves, too. We danced our way through most of the thirty-nine countries we visited."

Numerous fitness associations offer evidence that men who conduct symphony orchestras are among those who enjoy the longest, healthiest lives. It's all the upper-body aerobics involved in conducting, plus the power of command and the love of music. In my anecdotal findings, among those women who enjoy the longest, healthiest lives are those who do partner dancing. Maybe it's not a coincidence. Even as they are motivated to do far more exercise than most of their peers, their dancing also offers the satisfaction of even more basic needs among women. Despite the fact that they may be widowed and without the interest or opportunity to pair off again, they crave sociability, touching, laughter, and the male-female connection. As Dee Williams says, "You're partnering to do something as well as you can. It's that interaction that allows both the male and the female to relax and be themselves."

Doing a Hundred

The fastest-growing segment of the American population is people over 100. The second fastest is people who have passed the age of 85. This population tsunami of advanced seasoned women and men will only swell, driven by baby boomers, who have the good fortune of unprecedented levels of education and income, a keen awareness of good health habits, and access to cutting-edge medical resources. From the total of 70 million boomers born between 1946 and 1964, the MacArthur Foundation studies predict that approximately 3 million will live to the age of 100 or more.

Will you be one of them?

Centenarians live in a different dimension from the rest of us. Younger people are fond of saying "I need my own space." They are focused on how much square footage of living space they can afford, the height they intend to reach on their career ladders, the width of their social circle, and the dimensions of their bodies.

These are measurements that make up space—length, height, and width—the first three dimensions. What they leave out is the fourth dimension: time. However, objects exist in time as well as space (Einstein, of course, made this point in his theory of relativity). People, too, move across time as well as space. As Mai, the Santa Fe jewelry designer, said, "You're re-creating your reality as you move along through time and space—you're always designing."

Women and men who have successfully negotiated the passages of life may have accrued positive personality strengths, over time, that can carry them beyond their expected limits of physical strength and endurance. We see only the end result, the final effect, and not the causes that led to their extended life span.

Those who move beyond their eighties exist in a realm of time that is probably beyond the understanding of the rest of us—what I'll call the Fourth Dimension. Their space may be limited, since the majority live in retirement or nursing homes, or assisted-living facilities. They don't move around a great deal. The heights of their careers are well behind them; their social circles have contracted; and their bodies have shrunk. But where they expand beyond the rest of us is in the temporal dimension.

Centenarians are more focused on the present. They don't stress over things as much as the average person; they don't dwell on past mistakes or even potential future problems, including aging. "They manage their stress very efficiently," writes Dr. Thomas Perls, an associate professor of medicine at Harvard Medical School and director of the New England Centenarian Study (NECS). Fifteen hundred families have participated in the research study to date. When Dr. Perls applied a personality assessment tool to his subjects, he was most impressed with how low the centenarians scored on negative emotions—notably depression, anxiety, hostility, and social unease. High anxiety levels, he points out, disturb heartbeat, immune function, and blood clotting in ways that increase the likelihood of a heart attack. Some researchers believe these "aging accelerators" actually contribute to shrinking the part of the brain responsible for memory, which could hasten dementia.

Centenarians, by contrast, tend to be optimistic and able to live in the moment. A common attitude is "I just accept my life day by day." But they don't just sit back and passively accept losing out on activities or affection. They are active Seekers. The vast majority of the 330 centenarians actively participating in the NECS research in 2005 were alone, having lost their spouses, but 95 percent of them remain close with their families. The researchers say that staying involved with their family's lives is an important factor in allowing them to age successfully.

Sarah Weintraub speaks for many Seekers living in the fourth dimension. "I've done many things, I've been around the world, and I've loved many men," the 92-year-old said in a CNN interview. Asked to what she attributed her long life, she added, "I go to parties, weddings, bar mitzvahs—my family knows all they have to do is invite me and I'll show up. Sometimes they don't even have to invite me!"

This is what I mean by actively seeking engagement and attention. "The older people become, the more they are shunned by society," observes Lynn Adler, an Arizona attorney who has devoted much of the last twenty years to studying centenarians. "We all like attention, women and men, we don't outgrow that," she points out. "If it is hard to get a compliment at sixty, it's nearly impossible at a hundred. It's not easy to make ourselves pretty every day; it takes a lot of time, effort, and motivation. What is it that gives some people that inner motivation?"

One possible answer is a key quality of many centenarians: they are quick to be able to make an emotional connection with others. Think of Emily Anne and Gedney Tuttle, the widowed pair who were able to connect and fall in love in their late sixties; and Anna the Vamp of Tarzana, who in her seventies keeps boyfriends coming back to enjoy her companionship; and Kitty Hart, who, in her nineties, rotates among three suitors.

The Gift of Connecting

All humans are born with what medicine calls "limbic resonance," meaning the ability to tune in to the emotions of other humans. Women's brains are particularly hardwired with this capacity, most likely because a mother needs to be able to assess the internal state of a defenseless infant in order to respond appropriately. But as we move away from the mother-infant bond and conform to codes of behavior rewarded by our culture, many men and women allow this capacity to languish. Although the need to connect emotionally with others resurfaces for many women in their senior years, prompting them to reach out and help the defenseless, others grow inward and detach from their emotions, perhaps as a defense against their sorrows over losing loved ones and their sense of becoming invisible.

The "dazzlers" among seasoned sirens do not allow themselves to become invisible; they *command* attention.

I had hoped to question women nearing 100 about the need for intimacy even at advanced ages, and what one does about it. I approached the New England Centenarian Study to ask if I could interview some of their subjects. JaeMi Pennington, the community and media liaison, told me, somewhat abashedly, that the study does not ask questions about love or sex. But as a private citizen, he gave me a lead.

"Gramma's got a boyfriend," JaeMi had heard from his father several years ago. He had seen for himself when the family convened at Gramma's in Florida to celebrate her ninetieth birthday. "She couldn't keep it secret any longer," he told me, approvingly. "Both of them have lived long and happy lives with their families, and they are both very conservative. The nice thing is, he's not trying to be anyone's grandfather, or a stepdad, he's just trying to be my grandmother's boyfriend. There are no public displays of affection, but anyone can see they are unmistakably in love." I arranged to meet with Mrs. Pennington.

Seasoned Love Is Blind

The driver for Freedom Village is waiting for me at the baggage claim at Tampa Airport. He is accustomed to ferrying the residents of the retirement village to theaters and restaurants in Sarasota. He guesses that their median age is about 85.

"Are you visiting someone?" he inquires.

"Yes, a ninety-four-year-old woman and her eighty-nine-year-old boyfriend."

He chuckles. "That's it—the women like the younger men."

◆   ◆   ◆

"I'll meet you in the lobby, I'm wearing black and white." It's the bright voice of Catherine Pennington over the house phone. "Can I bring a friend to lunch?"

When she appears with her "friend," he and she are pushing a single stroller-walker with their arms entwined, her inside hand clasped over his. The scent of Chanel No. 5 precedes Catherine, a small, upright figure framed by a froth of snow white hair. She is wearing a print shirt over a white shell, white pants, and white ballet slippers. Her face is alive with expression.

She introduces her friend, an old-school gentleman by the name of Ward Luther. We cross a glass-enclosed bridge over a pond to one of the village's restaurants. Freedom Village is a fifteen-acre campus with six hundred residents spread out in three independent-living apartment buildings, but everyone seems to know Catherine and stops to chat with her.

"K-K-K-Katie, hello!" sings a man who passes us.

Catherine recognizes all of them by their voices or their silhouettes, or just by the way they carry themselves. Her lips are settled into a more or less perpetual smile, accentuated with bright red lipstick that she refreshes, reaching into the tray on the stroller and, with three quick swipes, precisely outlining her lips. "I still see my hair as auburn," she says, laughing at herself.

One would not guess that Catherine is nearly sightless. Several years ago she underwent eye surgery for macular degeneration. The surgeon did not notice that she was on a blood-thinning medication. Her eyes blooded during surgery, and she awoke functionally blind. She never gave a thought to suing. Nor has she let that life accident hold her back.

"I can see my hand, but I can't see my watch," she says, demonstrating how her watch "talks." When she is told she has a phone call, she does not use the stroller; she walks smartly to the dining room extension.

"But you didn't take the stroller," I say when she returns.

Catherine raises her fists and shakes them, her teeth clenched like a terrier, demonstrating the willpower that propels her.

I compliment her on her unusual earrings, long, gold filigreed hieroglyphs. "These are my Cleopatra earrings," she says proudly. "My son brought them to me from Egypt. He didn't have time to have them made up in my own name, but Cleopatra will do fine."

As I get to know this woman who is able to transcend human frailties and see beyond, it becomes clear to me that Catherine has a third eye. She can recognize friends. She looks directly at Ward, or at me, as if she sees us, and in a sense, she does. She also sees herself mirrored as an auburn-haired Cleopatra, which is not a bad self-image.

As she spoke, I learned that Catherine is not unlike her own grandmother, another dazzler who wore a huge diamond brooch fastened to her high lace collar. She, too, led several lives, traveling by covered wagon from Mississippi to Illinois to accept the proposal of a widower with four grown sons. She lived to the age of 95.

Catherine has no evident osteoporosis or trouble with arthritis. Her teeth are her own, minus a couple. And neither she nor Ward wears a hearing aid. I feel as if I'm talking to people somewhere closer to 70. Given that Catherine's younger friend is a handsome man, six foot–plus and remarkably fit for his nearly 90 years, I suggest that he must have been in the sights of many a lady in a retirement village where the women outnumber the men by ten to one. Why, then, was he attracted to Catherine, a widow five years older than he?

"She's different," says Ward. "Catherine has a little pepper in her. Good sense of humor. She thinks. And she talks a lot, so I don't have to."

Catherine loves sharing her vivid memories of growing up in Arcola, Illinois, a tiny farming town with brick streets, three banks, a hardware store, an ice cream parlor, a post office, and, believe it or not, an opera house. Born in 1911, before TV, psychotherapy, and superhighways, Catherine learned how to entertain herself, rely on herself, and lick her own wounds. She, her sister, and two mischievous brothers amused themselves by tying tin cans together and hiding in the bushes until a car came by, whereupon they would lasso a wheel and let the car dangle the clattering cans.

"We were devils," she says with pride.

She taught herself to drive at the age of 12 in her father's Model T Ford, secretly using a hairpin instead of a key to start it and careening down the closest alley. When her father finally caught her, he lowered the seat so she could reach the pedals. Her father was different, too. Pop was a wildcatter, always moving around the West looking for oil. Mother was a milliner who made all of Catherine's clothes and taught her to love to sew.

The memories she dwells upon are all happy ones: the high school summers when she and her friends would go to county fairs to dance to big-name bands like Benny Goodman's and Ozzie Nelson's, the train rides with Pop and her sister all the way to Chicago, where the girls could get their hair done and a first-class manicure. "Pop always said a woman owes it to herself to look the best she can," she says, extending fingers that are freshly polished and startlingly absent arthritic bulbs. Even setbacks are recast by Catherine with a silver lining. She had been accepted at college, but she had the misfortune of graduating from high school in

1929, when Pop saw his savings wiped out in the stock market crash. "Sorry, but I can't afford to send you away," he told her. But he would let her attend the nearby teachers' college.

"I won't be a teacher!" she resisted.

"Then you can just keep your job," he said.

She didn't complain. As a cashier at the local movie house, she was proud of earning her own good money—$15 a week. There were free mornings to play golf and dances to go to after the last picture show. When a barnstorming plane came through town, she thrilled to hedge-hopping up and down over the farm fences.

A college boy named Bower Pennington gave her a rush. He took her to the Indianapolis races and married her on election day of 1933, which saw Prohibition repealed and Fiorello La Guardia elected mayor of New York, a celebratory day all around. Their reception luncheon was held at the only eating place in town, Bucklermore Cafeteria. They honey-mooned all along the drive to New Jersey, where Bower had a job with Prudential Insurance Company. Catherine got her driver's license there at 22, a formality for which she had seen no need in her previous full decade of driving. She volunteered as a driver for the Red Cross and loved driving for a total of almost seventy years, until her husband retired and they moved to Florida and her eyes began to go.

She was 79 when her husband died in 1990. Catherine lived on in their Florida house by herself for a full year before making any decisions. She spurned offers from her four children to move in with one of them, instead putting her name on the waiting list at Freedom Village. One Friday she got a call that an apartment had suddenly come available, but she had to decide by Monday. Over that weekend she found a buyer for her house and moved on to her next life. No looking back.

"I talk a lot about the past," she tells me, "but I focus on the present."

❖   ❖   ❖

Catherine and Ward don't have to discuss the lunch menu. They know they will share a Reuben sandwich. When I ask them how long they have been coupled, there is a long pause.

"I don't even know how it started," says Catherine, purposefully vague.

Ward says, "It seems to me we go way back."

They eventually agree that they go back about thirteen or four-teen years. Ward tells me he is a descendant of Martin Luther's brother. A former engineer, he has been married twice and has three great-grandchildren, for whom he is writing a family history. His second wife died only two years after they moved into Freedom Village. He was des-perate for someone to talk to and do things with, but the male popula-tion of the place, already a distinct minority, kept dying off. Fearing that the ecological balance was at a tipping point, toward total domination by the female species, Ward and a few friends formed a dinner club called the Yellow Jackets. "We were making a statement: we may be the minority, but we can still be independent!" At the end of the year, the Yellow Jack-ets threw a party for the ladies. That's when Ward discovered that Cath-erine was "a lady of conversation."

She was also a big shot, he says—she was president of the residents' council and she called bingo at Freedom Village. So Ward joined the coun-cil and the bingo group. Then Catherine lured him back into engagement with their community by asking him to accompany her on her weekly visits to patients in the nursing home who were without family. That gave him the opening to invite Catherine to go out with him in his car to Sara-sota.

"It started with a few dates and grew and grew, and pretty soon I was getting fond of her," he says, at pains to impress upon me that there was "nothing flashy" about their romance.

Catherine's memory of their most romantic date was one Christmas when they attended midnight Mass together. "I was holding his arm. He put down his cane and fell over on the lawn, and I fell right on top of him!" she trills. "We went down in a heap, and neither of us could get up. So we lay there laughing."

"It just grew," says Ward.

"People began expecting us to be together," adds Catherine.

"But we created that impression."

He got her excited about dressing up in outlandish costumes for the monthly bistro nights. For the Oriental Bistro, Ward was austere in a Japanese kimono and Catherine majestic in a white silk Korean robe, given to her by her Korean daughter-in-law. They went bawdy for the

Western Bistro, with Catherine as a "madam" draped in a red feather boa on the arm of her "cowboy." For the Halloween party they went plain nuts, appearing as purple-haired punk skeletons.

They became so popular as a couple that on Valentine's Day 2002 the residents elected them "king" and "queen."

Although they spend just about every waking moment together, they keep separate apartments. They're smart enough to realize that they have very different tastes. Catherine's place is a backdrop for the treasured artifacts of her earlier family life: the antique silver service, the crystal decanters, her homemade lamps and needlepointed cushions, and walls of photos of her grandkids and great-grandkids. Ward calls his apartment "my bachelor pad"; there the furnishings are spare and as straight-lined as an engineer's blueprints, with dark leather chairs and a computer in the bedroom.

"We couldn't afford to get married," says Catherine. "I'd lose my husband's pension and my medical insurance. And without marriage, there's no sex involved," she volunteers.

"No question about sex," affirms Ward.

"He gives me a hug and a kiss when he leaves at night. And that's only happened in the last couple of years, right, Ward?"

"Uh-huh."

Catherine laughs and moves closer to me. "True confessions. I never went to bed with more than one man in my whole life—my husband. It's the way I was brought up."

"My upbringing was pretty much the same," Ward says.

The subtext in this conversation is that these two people are still ruled by the social restraints of their generation, even though they acknowledge that "our children have never asked."

"We're very attached," Ward offers with a tremor of deep feeling.

"Without Ward," Catherine says, "I'd be lost." She smiles slyly. "Plus I like him. I hope he likes me."

"Why do you think I stick around?"

While Catherine prepares a small cocktail party, Ward invites me to see his bachelor pad. He shows me the lengthy taped interview he has done of Catherine's memories. He draws an important distinction in acknowledgment of Catherine's pride of independence: "I am not her caregiver. I *care* for her."

True to the Sexual Diamond theory, he is now the nurturer, she the nurtured. Ward knows exactly how she likes her Canadian Club and soda fixed. They save their half-finished drinks until after dinner, then sweeten them up while they watch *The NewsHour* on PBS, after which Ward reads the newspaper to Catherine. She doesn't cook; she's had enough of that for one lifetime. Ward cooks, after a fashion, and they often have snacks in his apartment while he watches and she listens to their favorite baseball team, the Tampa Bay Devil Rays, lose again. If Catherine falls when climbing into bed, she has only to phone Ward and he'll pull on his pants over his pajamas, come up to lift her back into bed, and stay the night in her recliner.

◆   ◆   ◆

Even as we spend the day talking, the news is full of alarums about the impending doom of Hurricane Dennis, expected to hammer the Florida panhandle starting in forty-eight hours. "Are you worried?" I ask Catherine.

She tosses her hand toward the window. "You can't worry about stuff you can't do anything about—I've always been that way." She looks at Ward and laughs, offering her cheerful memory of hunkering down for the vicious Hurricane Ivan.

"I bought a sheer blue nightgown and matching peignoir. I thought I'd give Ward a shock if he stayed over!" She giggles. "But the lights went out, and we never got out of our clothes."

After a full dinner, I ask Catherine, "Does love make you stronger?"

"No question," she says.

Ward's love, transmitted not through words but through pure devotion, has carried Catherine over the threshold from sightedness to darkness without missing a day of laughter, or her après-dinner drink. And Ward has clearly found a new purpose in life in caring for her. He acknowledges it: "I think it's very important when you go to sleep at night to have something specific to look forward to the next morning."

Catherine Pennington is my vision of the fully seasoned woman. Peppery and sweet. Cleopatra and Grandma. Loving and beloved. She illuminates the Passage to Cultivation or Isolation described much earlier in this book. Resisting isolation, she turned over the soil in which she had lived with her husband, and soon after his death she cultivated a new community of friends and meaningful activities. Because she was doing what she loves, love found her, again. She retains strong ties with her own family and is nurtured by the acceptance of Ward's nearby children.

Her courage and feistiness in compensating for blindness have allowed her to reach an even higher state of mind. It is out of her physical affliction that she has cultivated second sight, the enlightenment to see past, present, and future more broadly, and to bless her own life history as happy and worthwhile. She fears death "only slightly." Her main feeling is that it's still so wonderful to wake up to the mornings; when her time comes, she will hate to miss it.

When her talking watch announces eight P.M., I suggest it's time to say good-bye. Catherine and Ward are reluctant—but the truth is, they've tired me out! They walk me to the elevator. I wait and watch as they turn and push the single stroller-walker together, arms entwined, her inside hand clasped over his. Two souls in resonance, moving as one.

Sex may be the last to go. But there is one thing that *never* goes—the only meaning that survives all—love.

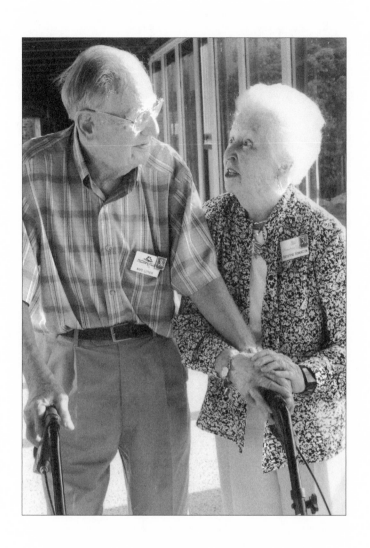

Appendix

This is the original questionnaire used in my research.

Welcome . . .

I am researching women's attitudes toward love, sex, dating, and new dreams over 50. Already nearly eight hundred women have responded to this survey. Please join in by answering the few questions below, and then tell us what you *really* think in the space provided. No need to give your name, but do give your e-mail address so I may contact you with invitations in the future.

After you complete the survey, hit SUBMIT and you'll go to the Seasoned Women's Network page, where you can read our current blogs and join in the conversation on our message board.

Thanks for your contribution.

Best wishes, Gail Sheehy . . .

Your age group:

- ○ 45–50
- ○ 50–55
- ○ 55–60
- ○ 60–70
- ○ 70–80
- ○ 80+

Your current relationship status? (Check all that apply.)

- ○ Married
- ○ Divorced or separated
- ○ Co-habitating
- ○ Widowed
- ○ Dating
- ○ Lover
- ○ Lesbian with partner
- ○ Lesbian without partner
- ○ Never married

Where do you live?

What car do you drive?

Where do you go for summer vacation?

Do you work?

- ○ Full-time
- ○ Part-time
- ○ Self-employed
- ○ Volunteer

How do you feel about sex over 50?

- ○ Hungry
- ○ Passionately enjoying it with a lover/lovers
- ○ Oh, I remember that
- ○ Never give up
- ○ Been there, done that, have other interests now

How do you feel about dating over 50?

- ○ Enjoying it
- ○ Actively seeking company
- ○ Wishful but too shy
- ○ Wish I could but I'm married
- ○ Revolted by the idea

What are you looking for in dating over 50?

- ○ Fun and companionship
- ○ Good sex
- ○ Possible mate
- ○ Sharing practicalities
- ○ A walker

Which man is more appealing to you:

- ○ He's younger, better in bed, and you can remain independent
  OR
- ○ He's older, slower, but he "gets you" warts and all

Are you tempted to have a love affair with a younger man?

- ○ Tempted, yes
- ○ Tried it and loved it
- ○ Tried it, and sorry I did
- ○ Not tempted

Have you noticed changes in your sexual desire or response with menopause?

- ○ No changes
- ○ Changes caught me by surprise
- ○ Lowered libido
- ○ Lowered energy
- ○ Pain with intercourse

My antidote for changes with menopause is:

- ○ New lover or new marriage
- ○ Novelties introduced in existing marriage
- ○ Hormones or vaginal estrogen
- ○ Self-stimulation
- ○ Grin and bear it
- ○ Gave up on sex

Now tell me what you really think:

Please submit your e-mail address

Acknowledgments

Writing is of necessity a solitary practice. But with this book I was surrounded by a "Team Sheehy" of such dedication and multiple talents that I never felt alone. Acknowledgment by name would not do justice to their pizzazz, nor would it show the spectrum of ages that became animated by this subject—from the twenties to the sixties.

My indefatigable editor, Monika Bauerlein, responded to my drafts straight through her pregnancy and delivery, as you can see from the photograph of Monika at her computer with baby Tonia at the keyboard. My two editorial assistants, Miranda McCloud and Kate Sweeney, gave daily, sometimes nightly, of their multiple skills and boundless enthusiasm.

Pat Allen, my dear friend and a visionary gynecologist, contributed from her vast experience in caring for this age group. Isatou Sawaneh brought an African perspective and kept us all organized. My brilliant website designers, Dave Campbell and Patrick Curran from 3 Rings Media, brought a welcome male perspective, as did director/photographer Vic Losick.

The group photograph could not include others who were also of primary importance in bringing the work to fruition. The Random House team: editors Jennifer Hershey and Laura Ford; executive publicity director Carol Schneider; marketing director Sanyu Dillon; and publisher Gina Centrello and associate publisher Libby McGuire. Dr. Melanie Horn, another dear friend and a wise West Coast psychologist, worked with me on some of the group interviews. Sarah Broom helped with logistics and setting up interviews.

Thanks are also due for the sustaining support of my agent, Amanda Urban; my legal adviser, Theodore Kheel; Surrendra Patel; Lai Chao; Yolanda Ormaza; and, as always, my husband and in-house editor, Clay Felker.

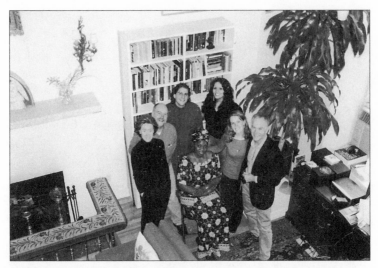

Team Sheehy. Standing, left to right: Pat Allen, Dave Campbell, Pat Curran, Miranda McCloud, Kate Sweeney, and Vic Losick. Seated: Isatou Sawaneh.

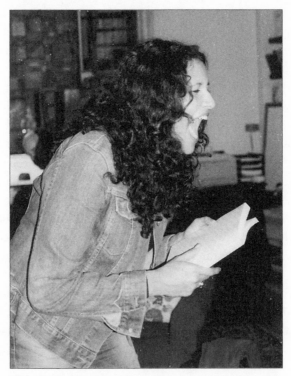

Miranda McCloud.

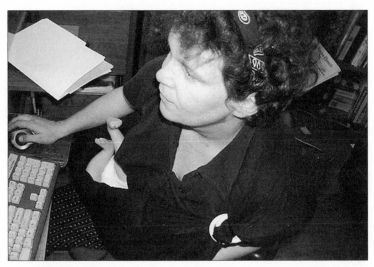

Monika Bauerlein.

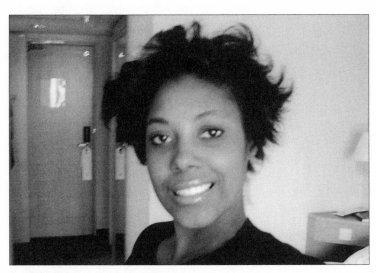

Sarah Broom.

Index

About the Author

Millions of readers around the world have defined their lives through GAIL SHEEHY's landmark work *Passages* and have followed her continuing examination of the stages of adult life in her best-sellers *The Silent Passage, New Passages,* and *Understanding Men's Passages. Sex and the Seasoned Woman* is her fifteenth book. Sheehy is also a contributing editor to *Vanity Fair* and a playwright. The mother of two daughters, she lives with her husband, Clay Felker, between New York and California. You can visit her at www.gailsheehy.com, and join the conversation on her newest website–blog–message board—Seasoned Women's Network.

About the Type

This book was set in Times Roman, designed by Stanley Morrison specifically for *The Times* of London. The typeface was introduced in the newspaper in 1932. Times Roman has had its greatest success in the United States as a book and commercial typeface, rather than one used in newspapers.